The Worry-Go-Round

by Melanie Cross

Published by:
Chipmukapublishing
PO Box 6872
Brentwood
Essex
CM13 1ZT
United Kingdom

http://www.chipmunkapublishing.com

Copyright © 2005 Melanie Cross

Proof-read by Nicholas Barrett & Anthony Griffiths

ISBN 1 905610998

AUTHOR'S NOTE

I wrote my book *The Worry-Go-Round* after suffering severe depressive illness in 1999. I was following a feeling that I 'just had to do it'. It wasn't as a form of therapy, it wasn't to massage my ego, and it wasn't as a form of 'revenge' on those whose actions had contributed to my breakdown. I wrote it for one reason, and one reason only; to help. To help those who were suffering or who had suffered from depression to understand their illness; to help those who were heading towards it to reassess their lives and see how they could change themselves and things around them; and to help the relatives and friends of people who were suffering to truly understand the pain, confusion, blackness and isolation in which their loved ones were immersed.

Depression is one of the last taboos. It is seen as a weakness, a flaw of character, something to be hidden from others and not talked about, which is why I wanted to help. I wanted to write a book to bring this illness into the open, for it to be discussed and for people to realize it is suffered by 'normal' people living 'normal' lives. I wanted to encourage people to seek help when they were distressed and feeling low, rather than wait until severe depression had them in its vice-like grip.

It was hard to revisit my long period of depression and write about my experiences, situations and feelings which had contributed to me being ill. I had long since left them all behind, but I knew that if I didn't write them down soon the memories would begin to fade of the life I had and the person I used to be. The identities and details of the characters in the book have been changed out of respect and privacy for those involved. People ask me if I am angry or hate some of the people who have been part of my life. I say no to both questions. Holding anger in your heart rots away your insides and makes you ill, and hate is also an ugly thing. I wish nothing but love to everyone that has been a part of my life; we all have our own lessons to learn and our own paths to follow. So I wish them good luck on their journeys also. Without them I would not have learnt so much and I would not be the person that I am today.

I hope people read the book and then look at their own lives. Maybe there are things they can change about their lives, their relationships, their situations and their own way of thinking in order to improve their lives and ultimately make them happier. Everyone deserves happiness; convincing yourself that you do is a hard thing. Once you believe you deserve to be happy you can begin to look at yourself and find your own 'truth'. When you have done this be true to yourself and follow your own true path. No-one can help you or tell you what it is; it is for you to rediscover the shiny bright thing that is you. Once you have done this protect it as it is the most precious thing in the world.

Finally I would like to say 'Thank you'. Thank you to all of my friends who were there for me and who have always been there for me; you know who you are.

Thank you to my parents for their unwavering support and endless love without which I would not be here today.

And lastly to my wonderful husband for his love, encouragement, understanding and for all of the help that he gave me in compiling this book.

Melanie Cross

FOREWORD

There's an old saying that I keep hearing. I've heard it used about children, life in general but mostly with regard to women - "they don't come with a manual, you know". Well, mine did.

When I first met Melanie she was working at the kennels and cattery mentioned towards the end of this book. She was every inch the healthy outdoor girl; fit, tanned, beautiful and very much in charge of her life. I couldn't reconcile this vision of contentment with the muttered advice my friend had given me - "she's lovely but, be careful, she's just recovering from a nervous breakdown". I simply couldn't imagine anyone less likely to have had a nervous breakdown - whatever one of those is.

We got on well, began stepping out together and the relationship grew. In time it became more serious and, after about eighteen months, we moved into a pretty Cotswold cottage together. Her job at the kennels had involved living in, so this meant a new job as well as a new home; a bit of a wrench perhaps, but maybe it was time to move on anyway. It was then she announced that she wanted to write a book.

She told me briefly what it was about and set to work. Although it sounded interesting I have to admit I thought her enthusiasm would wane and that in a few weeks she would be looking for something else to do.

Five months later the book was complete. Nine to five, six days a week, no breaks, no pauses, no doubts. Seldom have I seen such single-minded determination. And as for getting it published, have you ever tried sending a book, unsolicited, to a publisher? No? Well you surprise me. The world and his wife seem to be having a go. But it didn't faze Melanie one bit, she just kept on pushing until finally a door opened.

Reading the book I was struck by several things. The first was how powerfully she had described the feelings and emotions of someone plunging into the depths of depression. So powerfully that even an insensitive numbskull like me can understand them. Blackness, ugliness, unworthiness. The brittle veneer of happiness. It made me think, how many times have I heard the shrill overcompensating laughter of someone scrabbling for a grip on their lives and not realised how close they were to the edge? Maybe I'd even felt a bit like that myself on occasions, then through some lucky change in circumstance, had come back from the brink of the precipice without even realising I'd been there.

The second was how the events that pushed Melanie over the edge and into depression were just so normal. Distressing though it is, most people lose a grandparent, a pet, a job or a lover at some point in their lives. It's not as if she'd been cruelly disfigured in a freak accident, or taken hostage by terrorists, or spent her early childhood evading the Nazis. She's never done drugs, stolen a car, been arrested, or even been in a fight and thrown out of a pub (as far as I know). Melanie is a moderate person who was living a thoroughly normal life, just like me and, probably, just like you. But she still became ill. It really can happen to anyone. You can never say "I'm not the type".

The last thing that struck me was how arduous it was to recover so completely. Melanie had to question and confront and restructure so many aspects of her self. We all have so many built-in assumptions about what we should do with our lives, and expectations that we feel we should meet. And do we ever really consider whether they are right for us? The outer carapace that we present to the world doesn't have to change that much - certainly Melanie seems pretty normal most of the time, she watches soaps, curses other motorists and succumbs to the occasional fried breakfast - but now there's a steel core that simply will not allow a destructively stressful situation to develop. One of her rules is: if an issue keeps her awake at night she will resolve it the next day, no matter what it takes.

Some of my friends have asked me how I feel about the book being published. The answer is pride. Pride at the book itself and how she wrote it, pride at the way she endured her illness and recovered from it and pride at the help the book can give to those who read it. Look around you at your family, your friends and your work colleagues. Look at the person next to you on the bus or the train. Look at yourself. Learn to recognise the quiet cries and be ready.

James Cross BSc MSc PhD MIMechE CEng
Gloucestershire, UK
October 2005

CHAPTER ONE

The day that I finally broke down I remember huge thunderous teardrops thrashing silently onto the windowpane. They only whispered as they sleekly slithered their silvery snakes down to the sill, where they plopped in a pile and huddled together. The sky was pyre-grey and windily wild, shaking the trees angrily. I wasn't sure quite what they had done wrong, but Mr Wind had lost his temper so someone had to get it.

I sat dumbly in my chair, eyes squinting, trying desperately to focus on the raindrops, the trees, the forty small goggly-boggly eyes darting nervously in my direction. In fact anything swinging into focus would have made me feel a little more at ease. As it was, I thought my world was about to implode and leave a little black mark showing where I used to be. But the goggly-boggly eyes just kept on staring. They were no fools; they all knew that something was not quite right. A bit like an animal's sixth sense I suppose. Like on a volcanic island, when they all run into the sea and drown, just before she 'blows a big one'.

I had struggled on, feet of clay, on and on and on, dragging and dragging. Trying with every ounce of energy I had in my poor, sad, pathetic being to keep going. Not to give up, whatever life had to regurgitate and throw at me. But on that grey and dangerously menacing day, my soul and brain had been in conference together, and they had decided that enough was enough. This was the day that they had collaborated and decided they were going to shut down in a very united and definite way, in order to give me the chance to save myself from a very ugly, untimely and poisonous end.

Bang. Shutters down. Closed.

The eyes carried on staring and staring, wondering what to make of 'Miss Williams's' odd demeanour. I tried to keep my composure as I sat bolt upright on my chair. My soul seemed to be drifting and slippery-sliding out of my body and forming a little dirty black puddle of me, on the floor, at my feet. A very unusual and disturbing out of body experience. I didn't remember reading anywhere about out of body experiences being so terrifying. I thought it was supposed to be beautifully euphoric as you drifted and danced towards the heavenly whiteness of death. I felt cheated. I couldn't even get dying right.

I was desperately trying to hold on, as the seams that had held me together for so long stretched and gapped and threatened to explode and scatter my stuffing all over the floor. I tightly gripped my neck with one hand, trying to keep my head from lolling from side to side, back and forth, a nodding dog in the back of a car. My grip tightened and my nails sunk further into my sensitive flesh, not only leaving moon symbols of my desperation, but giving slight physical pain to vaguely detract me from the emotional pain that I had been carrying for months, and when I honestly think about it, years. In fact, when I think back, I had been carrying emotional pain for as long as I could remember.

The hands on the clock seemed to quietly slide backwards that afternoon, and every minute seemed to trickle into an eternity. I couldn't give way to this intensity of feeling. I couldn't let go and allow myself to give in. Not until I had let the children go from my care and back into the safe arms of their parents, where their innocent hearts had not yet been victim to the cruelties of life.

When the bell for the end of the day finally decided to elude me no further and let its strangled chicken squawk echo around the building, I realised I had finally managed to claw myself to the end of the day. The relief I felt when the little sweethearts had been safely dispersed was immense. I now knew that if I collapsed and died on the floor, at least they would not have to be witness to it. They were safe.

I could feel the last droplets of energy slowly seeping from me and dribbling away as I grabbed my bag and coat and things that I needed to fruitlessly prepare for the following day. Rerunning the actions I had made so many times before. I thought if I kept some kind of normality and recognisable behaviour it might just override the wave after wave of distorted vision I was experiencing as I lapsed in and out of the waking coma. There was no thought as to what I had collected, no planning. I just squashed as much as I could carry into my plastic box and bulging bags and hoped in vain that I had something, anything, in there that may be of some use. How I managed to do this I will never know. So very pointless; a pointless empty gesture to myself that everything was okay and I was absolutely fine. Still not giving in. What a fool.

Going through the motions of normality held me together enough that day to help me get home. Going through the motions of normality was the very thing that had helped me keep going for this long, the thing that had helped me doggy paddle my way through the previous few months keeping my head only just above the murky water, saving me from sinking under the inky stillness, drowning and drowning and smiling my way into the welcome oblivion.

The rain thundered on the windscreen, and the wipers hypnotically swished wet rainbows through the persistent splattering. But still there was silence. There was an eerie lack of any noise at all that day. It had been like that all afternoon, an afternoon of my life in slow and noiseless motion. Maybe my brain had been saving its last pin head dribbles of energy to get me home, so it had turned off all unnecessary activity. Or maybe my terrified desperation had blanked out everything around me. Which ever it was, I found myself on the doorstep at home. Home to safety. Home to the last remaining sanctuary.

Bulging bags splayed on the step at my feet, and sodden clothes clung on in limp and lifeless desperation to the huddled wreckage that was me. I didn't bother trying to wrestle with the baggage in an attempt to find a key. I couldn't. I just couldn't. With my last dregs of energy I raised my icy fist and pounded the door. The silence still span around me, and my head began a dull and aching thud, thud, thud. The door swung open before me. A look of pale horror swept across my mother's face as I stepped over the heap of pointlessness at my feet and began to lurch up the stairs.

"I feel bad Mum....really bad," I whispered, as I collapsed my dirty, soggy body, still clothed and shoed between the fresh clean sheets. My contaminating ugliness began to seep out of me and soil the cleanliness enveloping me. My head began to crack and shatter with the all-consuming thumping thuds of unrelenting pain. My last drip of energy dribbled and dropped out of me along with the never ending icy tears which streaked my face. My body became heavy, and the broken pieces of my soul went slip sliding out of me and gathered in dirty darkness under the bed. My eyes cracked shut. I was gone. Shattered. Exploded. Extinct.

CHAPTER TWO

I really don't know how I did it, but I managed to go to school the next day and even taught all day. I phoned to make a doctor's appointment and went to see him after school. Driving there I felt a little nervous. I wasn't quite sure what to say, or how to tell him why I was there. I didn't know what was wrong and I didn't know how to explain myself. It wasn't like I had a rash or a lump or an unexplainable ache. There was nothing obviously wrong with me, and I was just being stupid. I was a time wasting fraud. The doctor would see right through me and see me for what I really was – a useless, dirty, black smudge. I sat in the waiting room trying to look normal, trying to look as if nothing was wrong with me. I thumbed pointlessly through magazine after magazine. Not reading a word, not looking at a picture, just thumbing and thumbing. I was trying so hard not to tap my hands or feet with nerves as my body quietly shook and my stomach held on to its solid churning knot of somersaulting nervousness. I could feel everyone's eyes boring into me, but I just couldn't look up and meet their stares. I felt too guilty. I could hear them silently screaming. They were screaming 'Fraud, fraud, fraud!' as I pushed myself further and further back into the chair, hoping no-one would notice me squirming there.

A voice broke the terror... "Rachael, come on in."

My mind swung back and focused on reality and I slid off of the chair like a snake's belly and slithered my way through the door after the doctor, droopy-shouldered and head hung low. I wanted to turn tail and run away and scream and scream. But I followed the doctor's gestures towards the black chair of judgement and slumped down. Not looking up, not looking anywhere.

"How can I help you?" he smiled. Christ!! How can you help? How can anyone help? My soul was screaming and screaming. 'I am a fraud. I have no right to be here. There are people who need you who are really ill. There is nothing wrong with me. Why am I here? I shouldn't be here, I am a fraud. I am a fraud. I am a fraud. I'm insane. I'm completely insane.' My head spun round and around and I wished the lights would black out and all this pain would end. For good. Forever.

I pulled myself up as straight and as tall as I could in the chair, swung my eyes up to meet the doctor's sympathetic gaze, and took a long deep breath.

"I'm really sorry to bother you, but I don't feel too good," a strange voice squeaked out,

"I can't go on any more."

"I feel like I'm going to die."

I was trying so hard to keep some kind of sane composure but my eyes began to betray me, and stinging tears washed down my face in an inconsolable waterfall of grief. I can't really remember what was said after that. I shook and cried and shook and cried and babbled on inanely with what I thought must have been very incoherent nonsense. To the doctor though I must have made some sort of sense. To him it must have been obvious, another textbook case.

We spoke for at least half an hour, but to me it seemed like a tiny speck of time. He asked me lots of questions that merged and blurred into each other, but there was one sentence that I remember vividly. It was the words that began the long and very painful journey of recovery.

"You are no longer in control of your life," he said slowly and meaningfully in order for my scrambled brain to digest it. How dare he! How dare he tell me I'm not in control, he must think I'm completely useless. A huge wave of anger, disbelief and resentment began to well up inside me, which was then washed away with the words that followed.

"You are no longer in control of your life. I am in control of your life. I am taking away your responsibility for yourself in order for you to have a chance to begin recovering. You need to rest, and you need to take time to resolve some of the things that are making you feel so bad. I'm not going to give you any antidepressants at the moment, but I am going to sign you off work for two weeks. This will take you up to the Easter holidays and enable you to have a break and a rest. Maybe you should think about whether you feel it would help you if you spoke to a counsellor, and come back in a week's time and let me know how you are feeling. If you need to see me before then or if you have any more thoughts of suicide please come back. I am always here."

An overwhelming feeling of relief swept over me. My whole being let out such a huge sigh of relief I was sure that everyone could hear it, and I wobbled out of the doctor's room like a wrung out dish cloth – limp, lifeless and soggy.

The doctor had told me I was not well. But I found it very hard to absorb this information. I didn't need counsellors, or pills, I just needed a rest…a good long rest. I was not a lunatic who needed to speak to anyone, that would show I was weak and unable to help myself. I was a bright, intelligent, outgoing, strong person. I didn't need anyone else's help. I would be fine. I didn't need pills. Pills were for losers, people that were weak and couldn't cope with the real world. I would be fine. I would be okay. There was nothing wrong with me. I would be fine. I would be fine.

CHAPTER THREE

Day after day smudged into one and I lay in bed. I lay in bed and slept and slept and slept. I'd heavily haul my huge lumpiness out of bed in the morning. But throughout the day the heavy head shutters slowly began to lower lead-like on to the top of my brain. My head would become heavier and heavier and my eyes dangled and drooped onto my cheeks. Wherever I was, what ever I was doing, I had to lie down and shut my eyes. Whether this was in the car, on the floor, or anywhere at all, I just had to do it. If I didn't lie down to rest and sleep and sleep and sleep I knew I would topple over and collapse. I had to lie down to relieve the heaviness inside my head. Every day I fought myself, and every day I lost. I tried. I tried really hard to beat it, but it always won.

'Sixteen hours sleep a day must be doing me good,' I thought. 'I must really need this rest... I'll be better soon.'

I couldn't go out anywhere where I knew I couldn't lay down. I was terrified. If I couldn't lie down I would collapse, and that was that. I didn't know what to do. I kept trying to reassure myself that I would soon be feeling like my old self again and that everything would be fine. Everything would be fine. Everything would be fine.

I began to think back to when I was feeling full of energy and on top of the world. Now when was that?... The black droplets of reality and realisation trickled into the little bit of my head that seemed to be working correctly. I couldn't remember the last time I had felt on top of the world. My energy had slowly been seeping away over the past ten months. When I really thought hard about it I realised, drip by drip, my life force had trickled away leaving me empty. I hadn't taken time to refuel. I hadn't taken time to give myself the essential things in life that one needs to keep going. No rest, no TLC, nothing in life that I wanted, never thinking of me. I had spent my whole life giving, giving, giving and everybody taking, taking, taking. I had been left with nothing – an empty husk of ash. One last little poke and I would crumble to the floor and float away in the breeze. The end.

I had been struggling for months with exhaustion and the relentless military monotony of every day life. The sparkle that I once had teaching had long since twinkled away leaving me battling with paperwork, bureaucracy, and bullshit. The whole purpose of teaching had gone, and I didn't want to be a secretary, baby sitter, whipping post. The tiredness had darkly tiptoed into my life and stretched its bony black fingers around me. Every day it gripped a little tighter, and a more and more gruelling struggle took place as I tried to survive each day. I would drag myself home and collapse under a pile of preparation, planning, and paperwork, then pour myself into bed. Every day became the same – harder and harder.

I smiled my way from behind my mask of control and calm, and the creeping cracks grew deeper behind it. I was sure no-one could see them. How clever I was. I was fooling them all. It didn't matter that I would crawl into the loos at lunchtime and silently scream and cry and cry to release the pressure that was about to make the top of my head explode and light up the sky like bonfire night. Letting the pain leak out quietly, that was the way. No-one would know.

Sometimes I walked the streets in the lunch hour releasing the same silent tears as my feet dragged through deadness of Autumn about my feet, and the grey drizzly puddles reflected my life back at me. But still my mask shone rosy cheeked, and no-one knew. Maybe if they had looked deep into my eyes, through the slits in the mask where my soul peeked out, they might have glimpsed the truth. But still no-one saw.

Sleep evaded me. The thing I needed most. Every night I would crumple into bed expecting to slip into sleep as my body and brain ached for rejuvenation. But every night I lay in the dark. Exhausted. Awake.

My mind and body that had so heavily sunk into the bed waited for the sleep switch to flick on, but it didn't. I would lay alone in the dark, alone in a world surrounded by people. The blackness entombed me, the whole world was gone, and I was alone with myself. The only person I had. The only person I didn't want to be with.

Then the worry-go-round would begin. It would start to spin slowly at first, but would then glide up to a speed that was a little too quick for me to jump off. The events, worries and fears that I had managed to suppress for the whole day would be splattered into my consciousness all at once.

"If you can't look at the grubby mess of your life during the day, then you will damn well have to face your demons at night," the darkness slyly sneered. And so the night-time battle would commence.

I tried everything. Warm baths, hot milk, reading, natural sleep remedies, but nothing would dampen down my brain's unwelcome night-time activity. I would lay in bed as each hour passed and try to dodge the undermining bombardment of fears, insecurities and unresolved mess that was my life. I tried to think of beautiful things, of loved ones, of happy times, but the worry-go-round would spin them off. "No room for you on this ride!" cackled the darkness. The black stallions bucked and kicked with nostrils flared and eyes glinting, until every white thought was gone, and I spun on the ride terrified and alone with the black beasts.

Sometimes I would slide into sleep as dawn's grey fingers poked through the curtains. Sometimes I would fall asleep as my head touched the pillow, only to wake up a couple of hours later to ride around and then sleep for an hour before I got up. Sometimes I would sleep until dawn, then wake up and ride around and around and around until I got up. The crumbs of sleep that I swept together were never enough to feed the tired exhaustion. As time went on I always awoke more tired than I had gone to bed, which made the days harder and harder to crawl through, and on and on it went.

'Exercise is the answer,' I thought. 'This will help me sleep. Exercise makes you look better, feel better, get fitter.' I hoped it would work.

I had gone to the gym for years and I had done every exercise class they had to offer. Every night after school I would go there for at least an hour to do some class or another. Whizzing and leaping and sprinting and sweating. I had lost a lot of weight, trimmed up, got fit, made friends, and it had been a life saver on many occasions.

'If you exercise you get more energy and it helps you sleep better,' I was always told. I found this to be true for many years but when I needed its help the most it began to become more and more difficult. The classes were great for forgetting for a brief moment in time all of the bad things, but they soon bounced back when the classes finished.

I had always left the gym feeling exhilarated, fit and happy, but this feeling became less and less frequent. It began to become a real struggle to go, a struggle to do the classes and a struggle to get home afterwards. Exhilaration was replaced with exhaustion, fitness with fatness and being happy with being sadly distraught. I kept trying to leap but limped, dance but dangled and prance but I plopped like a pebble in a pool where the ripples washed inwards and began to drown me.

Exercise had kept me going for a long time, but finally it was no longer any good for me. In fact it was hopelessly bad, so I stopped going.

As I began to feel worse another friend came to lend a hand, to make me feel better, sleep better, cope better. Bottle shaped and beautiful, whispering promises of seductive solace and brief relief; a little to have with dinner, a little to spend the evening with, a little to help me sleep; a little...only a little.

'A bottle of wine is fine,' I thought. 'One per night, all right then maybe two. It's not that bad. Sociable, that's what I am. A bit of comfort, surely that's not wrong. It might help me sleep and it's better than drugs from the doctor. I'm fine, really. It's just helping for a little while, blocking things out, a little relief; anything to help the pain. Surely that's okay,' I would tell myself.

I would drink with friends, I would drink with meals, I would drink watching television and I'd drink before I went to bed. A cool glass of wine in my hand was like a golden chalice holding a protective elixir, pure and beautiful. It was a magical potion but it never produced the same feelings each time it was administered for purely 'medicinal' reasons. Sometimes it picked me up, sometimes it brought me down, sometimes it helped me sleep, sometimes it didn't. Many times I drank until I couldn't see or think properly, and I'd incoherently talk to myself while mopping up the wine that seemed to be leaking from my eyes. No matter how it made me feel it was better than being left alone with the sober realities of life. Being drunk was better.

I remember sitting one February night in the chilly darkness of the garden accompanied by as many of my father's cans of lager as I could find. It must have been about 2.00am and everyone in the house was asleep. I sat and sat and sat, and drank and drank and drank, and cried and cried and cried, and stared at the stars waiting for an answer. But one never came. I sat until my T-shirt covered body was frozen, soaking and stiff. I drank until I couldn't see or feel or think. And I just cried. I knew something was wrong, terribly wrong, but I just didn't know what to do make things right.

I wasn't drinking so much now though. How could I when I was spending all of my time asleep? Things must be getting better I thought. I'll feel great soon and then I'll be fine to go back to school after Easter.

CHAPTER FOUR

Simon and I sat in the pub, my favourite place to be. I'd asked Simon to come with me as I didn't want to go on my own, mum said she would come but I didn't want to upset her any more than she had been. My mess. My problem. One large glass of wine for nerves, one for luck and one for the road, then off we went.

I couldn't face doing what I had to do, but it couldn't wait any longer. If I wanted to rest properly I had to begin to do the things that would help me rest a little easier, and this was one thing that I couldn't put off any more.

We stood outside the shop, my stomach churning and tears prickling the backs of my eyes.

'I am NOT going to cry,' I told myself sternly as I pushed open the door and stepped into a world of magic and make believe. A place where everything was beautiful and dreams came true. Dresses and gowns of lace and silk and satin shimmered and glimmered and danced out at me. Iridescent swathes of heavenly cloth hung like frosty flowers, fragrantly surreal. Tiaras and crowns of diamonds and pearls, gold and silver, bows and flowers, and fairies and towers, all burst forth from an explosion of someone's dreamy imagination. Hundreds of fairy tales were hanging there, just waiting to be kissed gently to life by love.

I didn't belong to this sparkling, romantic, white world. I never would. I was the dirty troll seeping out trails of dankness and infecting the fairy tales. I had to do this as quickly as I could, before I had time to think about what I was doing, and before I had time to contaminate anyone else's fairy tale.

I fastened the complicated arrangement of ribbons and buttons on my own as I didn't want anyone else to see me, and I shuffled out of the changing room apologetically. I was a grizzly grey gargoyle in a golden gown. It looked good. I did not.

"You look beautiful... If I wasn't married I'd marry you," Simon smiled. "He's a really, really stupid man."

He was so supportive, and so, so sweet.

I smiled back at him feeling like the fraudulent fake that I was.

"The wedding's off," I cheerfully told the assistant from behind the mask. "I've paid for the dress so I thought I'd better come and collect it."

Inside my edges were curling up with embarrassment. The shop assistant hopped from one foot to the other not quite knowing what to say at my apparent cheerfulness over such a rotten situation. If only she knew.

I took the dress off as quickly as I could because I didn't want my troll muck rotting it. I wasn't entirely sure what I was going to do with it, but I couldn't cope with any more smiley phone calls reminding me that I hadn't picked it up. The shop assistant wrapped it and packed it as quickly as she could as she just couldn't face me, and she knew that I just couldn't face her.

So relieved the ordeal was over, I struggled out of the shop with my cumbersome package, and when I got home I put it at the back of the cupboard in the darkness, out of reach, out of sight, alongside my dreams.

CHAPTER FIVE

I drove slowly to stop the plates of armour that I had bolted together from grinding and clanking. I was about to embark on my next mission and I knew he would be there, as he had to be, he had changed the locks; changed the locks with everything that I possessed inside. It was his last attempt to try and keep me in the prison of his tangled world. He was still in control, possessing the possessions, and he liked it that way. He wanted to keep me, so he had locked me in and locked me out.

Confusion. So much confusion.

I had discovered that he had changed the locks when I went to collect Sophie, my black much-loved cat. I had begged Guy to look after her for me for a little while, so that I could find her a new home; but he wouldn't, he hated her. He had always hated her. He hated everything that I loved and he had always tried to destroy anything and everything that I ever cared about. He was always shouting at her for going upstairs, shouting at her for sitting on the furniture, just shouting and shouting and shouting. He was good at that. His speciality you might say. He'd tease and torment her until she'd spend all of her time, day after day, curled up invisibly in her basket, flinching whenever he walked by. I knew how she felt. Her skin problems were made worse by stress so I had to bathe her three times a week in the sink to help to ease her discomfort. But that would make him shout more, which would make her scared more, and on and on it went – a circle of the vicious kind.

I couldn't leave her, I couldn't take her with me, I had to do what was best for her, and it broke my heart.

My mum and I turned up at the house that day, the cavalry with the cardboard carrier. The kind lady at the Cats Protection League was going to take her in and find her a nice new home, a much better home than I had given her. I was supposed to have looked after her and given her a new start in life, but I had failed miserably when I had moved in with Guy and brought her with me. She had spent the whole time terrified. We both had. What kind of awful mother had I been, cruelty by my own gutless inaction. I was such an ostrich, and I hated myself for it.

I tried to turn the key in the lock, but something was wrong, it was rigid. It wouldn't turn and it wouldn't budge. Cold fear and disbelief swept over me as I realised that I was locked out of what was supposed to be my house. My hands began to shake, as I really couldn't understand what on earth was going on. I had to get her, I didn't have a choice, and I was not going to leave her to be a victim of his own self-loathing, she deserved happiness, so much more happiness. I had let her down so badly that I hated myself for being so spinelessly pathetic, and it had to stop. It had to stop now.

I held open the cat flap and called her; if I couldn't get in she'd have to come out. I had been reduced to grovelling in the dirt, on my knees yet again, and the humiliation was unbearable. My mother sat tight lipped and tamping trying hard not to make things worse by telling me what she thought of him. I already knew what she thought of him. I knew what everyone thought of him.

When Sophie realised I was outside she came running out, tail in the air, and leapt into my arms. She was a little streak of sunshine cutting through the darkness. Her skin was weeping and her baldness was shining out in patches, but she didn't care she just purred and purred and nuzzled into me. So we took her away.

I had remained composed and calm until we arrived at the lady's house, then everything that I had held back rushed out in torrents. I was so ashamed and embarrassed. I explained that all of Sophie's toys and food, and bed and bowls and medication were locked in the house, and I couldn't get in and I was mad, mad, mad. I cried and cried and cried inconsolably. A shaking tree in a gale of anger and sorrow. I was so useless. Such a failure. I didn't deserve to have her, so now I was being punished for being the pathetic pile of uselessness that I was. How could I have let things get like this?

Sophie ate a little of the food in her cage and sat in the warm fluffy bed.

She smiled out at me. She was safe. "I'm going to be okay mummy. It's alright. Don't cry," she smiled and smiled and softly purred.

"I love you sweetheart. I'm so, so sorry. This is the best thing for you, and I love you so, so much, don't ever forget that."

My mum led me out. I couldn't see; my eyes were welded shut with tears. The lady reassured me everything would be okay, her aura glowed, and I believed her. But it didn't take away the sickness in my stomach, the anger in my head and the pain in my heart.

Now I was heading back for one last time, full of fear and dread. I didn't have the strength to collect my things but I knew I had to; I didn't have a choice. I had to go back just one last time, and I couldn't relax until I had. I had been worrying and worrying and I knew it just wouldn't go away until I had done it. So there I was dangling droopily on the doorstep surrounded by baggy, bedraggled boxes ready to pack my broken life into. Shaking and sickly scared I reached for the doorbell. He had to let me into the house as I knew I couldn't get in because of the locks. That was the only thing I did know. I didn't know who he was anymore, I didn't know who I was any more; I didn't know anything anymore.

The door swung open and the stranger stood there blank and unemotional. A cunning disguise for a seething sea of anger. I could feel my insides starting to crumble, and I could hardly stand up, as I dragged the boxes inside. He wouldn't help with the boxes but, bless him, he had started to help with my packing. There was a box of battered and torn books ready in the hallway, and a smashed and splintered pile of tapes and cases at the bottom of the stairs. Well it was quicker to throw them down the stairs than to carry them wasn't it. I quietly swept them into a box and sat in a putrid puddle of silent streaming tears on the kitchen floor. I crudely wrapped things in newspaper and stuffed them into boxes. I wanted to get out so fast that I only grabbed the things that I knew I must take, and then left the rest of my belongings. I really didn't care any more. I had lost my house, my furniture, my cat, my relationship, my health and my sanity, so to worry about a few pots and pans seemed so completely pointless it really didn't matter. Nothing mattered any more. I robotically wrapped things not knowing what I was doing or where things were going but I carried on. It was the only chance I had to scrape together what was left of my life, so that I could put it away somewhere safe until I was ready to face myself once more. As the tears rolled I sat and sobbed in piles of paper and pointless packing, praying for the pain to end. It must end. It had to end.

He stood and he watched. He stood and he watched, checking I wasn't taking anything I shouldn't. So much love, so much trust. He had everything, I had nothing, yet still he watched. I had been kicked and smashed and bashed and crushed until I didn't know which way was up and which way was down and which way was forward and which way was back. So I sat on my head, inside out. And still he watched.

"I still love you," said the stranger, as he stared black eyed and motionless.

I looked up with smudgy faced disbelief, open mouthed and withering. Does not compute. Does not compute. One last kick for old times' sake.

"You don't have to leave...I only broke your things because I was so angry and I wanted you to stay. I love you."

He had such special ways of showing his love.

If I could have risen from the floor, the place I belonged, I would have hit and smashed and bashed him, until finally he might just have felt a tiny piece of the pain he had given me to carry. But I couldn't, because he still held onto my strings – the most marvellous and magnificent puppeteer.

I dragged myself across the floor and disappeared. I drove away from everything, away, away, away, but not escaping.

I couldn't get out of bed for four days afterwards, but I was going to be okay soon. Okay. Okay.

CHAPTER SIX

Day after day passed by and I felt no better. I really couldn't understand it. I was so sure I would feel better after a rest, but it was just not happening. I was so angry with myself. I was so weak, so pathetic. The noose at the end of the Easter holidays was swinging in the breeze before me, taunting me, sizing me up, knowing I was on my way. I knew what it meant. I was terrified. If I couldn't get out of bed, how the hell was I going to do the 60-hour week of a teacher? I became more and more fearful as I was sucked down into the spiralling black hole. I must try to do something normal, something to help, I thought. If I pretend it's not happening it might just go away. Maybe it's all in my mind. So I decided to go out for the afternoon with some friends.

I spent two hours trying on clothes, trying desperately to find something that would make me look normal – a disguise. I loved fancy dress and now I was dressing up in a fancy dress disguise pretending to be me. No-one will notice if I do a really, really good job I thought. Everything I tried on was soiled with the sickening stench of memories. I couldn't escape them. They were dangling there for all to see and mock, mock, mock. Everything I tried was the same, so I put on something or another and patted and patted the clothes to try and bash some of the dangling dirt off. I looked at the reflection of my battered mask in the mirror. It was still hanging on in there. The creases and cracks underneath it had begun to rot their way to the surface, and it was beginning to splinter and flake and fall on the floor at my feet. I patched it as best I could with a trowel full of make up, and I worked really hard at the black pendulous bags which had bulged out from the mask and hung under my eyes hammock-like, begging for more sleep. I skilfully worked to hide the yellowy white troll juice, my complexion, which had now begun to leak out spreading all over the mask and drowning it. Blusher, blusher, blusher, I look normal now. I stood back to admire my skilful deception, and I was foolishly pleased with my results. So I propped up my mask, which was now threatening to slide down my face, and off I went.

We arrived at the psychic fair; here I would find some answers. As I walked into the large function room, my stomach was tied in knots, and the tape on my mask was peeling off each time I moved. In the middle of the room were large tables decked in purple velvet. They were covered in things to buy, things you needed, things to make you feel better. Books on visions, and angels, and psychic powers, and dowsing, and ghosts, and UFOs, and healing, the list was endless – books for all eventualities and predicaments. There were tarot cards to buy to tell you your fortune, but I didn't want those. There are only a certain number of times you can draw the crumbling tower and death. I had seen it all before.

I eyed the array of dazzlingly sparkly crystals that shone out like a hundred rainbow coloured stars, glittering and dancing. They mesmerised me and called me in. "Come closer," they whispered, "come closer." I slid towards them drawn by the sliver of beauty in the darkness. There were twinkling crystals for dowsing that gently swung on chains waiting to show people the way, or give them answers to those all-important questions.

"Choose me, choose me," they called. Below them in little wooden trays were crystals of every colour and they all claimed to help. Some were for health, some for wealth, some for love, some for joy. There was a crystal there for just about everything you might need one for, but not one for me. The young girl behind the table eyed me suspiciously. Her dark eyes darted from side to side like a nervous rat, and she was far too bony. Far too bony. Her clothes draped on her like a broom-handle scarecrow and lank straw clung to her forehead. She stared into my eyes. Spooked, I flapped my raven wings and was gone.

I pushed my way through the huddles of people, I could hear people talking and people laughing but they seemed a million miles away. A million miles away, but I could still feel their eyes as they whispered from behind their hands and mocked the troll. I could hear them. I could hear them. Around the edges of the room were small tables decked in an array of silks and satins and velvets. Upon the swathes of coloured cloths were crystals, feathers, pendants, tarot cards, golden angels, pictures, black cats and crystal balls. Each table looked different from the next, and each person sitting behind the tables looked different from the next. Some looked like witches and wizards, some looked like grannies and mums, some looked like hippies and gypsies, and they all looked normal and they all looked inside me. I could feel their eyes boring into me, and I realised to my horror that all of these people had the talent for looking behind the mask. They could all see me for who I really was – the troll. I could feel myself becoming more and more embarrassed, my legs began to shake, sweat trickled, my heart pounded, and I slumped in front of Patricia; I had come this far and I needed answers.

Her coal eyes lifted and looked deep into mine through her tangled, spidery, mascara choked eyelashes.

"You would like a reading?" she asked through smiles and her thick Brummie accent. Her tumbling earthy curls framed her wizened bronzed face. Her golden jewellery glittered in the mesmerising candle flickers and her smart suit gave nothing away of her ability as a medium or her psychic talents. She looked like a pub landlady. And boy I needed a drink.

She talked me through what she was going to do and how it worked and popped a tape into the recorder so that I could listen to what she had to say again, once I had got home. She got me to shuffle a pack of tarot cards which she said were an aid to helping her read me. I didn't think she needed them. I was spilling out all over the floor. She spoke to me for about forty minutes telling me what had gone, where I was now and where I was going. I tried hard to take it all in, but found it difficult, as my concentration span would not last for more than a minute at a time. I was glad she was taping it. She told me lots of things I knew to be true, but I know she saw a lot, lot more. She could see the torment and ugly demonic blackness that massed and swirled murkily underneath the mask and deep, deep inside me. But she said nothing. I knew she knew I was mad. But she said nothing. I was screaming and screaming inside, 'Say it! Say it! Say it!' but she said nothing. I was far too evil and frightening for her to tell me the truth. She must have been terrified. She carried on pretending I was normal, and the jumbly words kept tumbling out.

"Any questions?" she smiled.

Fumbling dumbly I mumbled no, paid my money and shuffled away with tape in hand.

The room swirled and faded in and out and in and out of focus. I felt the familiar feeling of my soul slipping and sliding in and out of my body. I fled from the room full of scornful, slitty eyes, and shaking and swaying bought a coffee and cake and crumbled into a chair. A coffee to keep my eyes from clamping shut and dragging me helplessly into sleepy oblivion, and cake, I hoped fruitlessly, would give me enough energy to get home. I couldn't leave; I had to wait for the others. Trembling, dribbling cake down my front, I wedged myself upright and tried with blood vessel bursting concentration to stop my eyes from rolling backwards and ceasing to work. I battled in the twilight zone with the enemy, which was me, and all around saw nothing. They chattered and nibbled and laughed, laughed, laughed. And I did battle with the blanket of darkness that was trying to smother and choke and black me out. And they carried on as if nothing was happening. No-one came to save me, no-one helped. They all laughed and mocked and sneered from behind their unaware normal exteriors.

The baking smoke choked me; slip sliding inside, I died.

I got home. I now believe in miracles.

I lay on the floor, unable to move, eyeing the chalk line around my body. I could see beside and all around a jigsaw of fragmented mask pieces, slimy, stinking, shattered. Unmendable. I tried to stretch my fingers out to sweep, sweep, sweep up the last splinters of security, but could not move. The mask was destroyed. There was nothing left except the pungent smell of decay as the rot seeped lead-like to the bottom of the carcass. It formed sticky pools of oily blackness deep inside, silently, slowly, still.

I was the naked troll.

No more hiding for you young lady. No more hiding for you. I was left with the one, the only thing in the world that I did not want. Me.

I tried in vain to lift my arms, my head, my legs. I tried and tried and tried to sit up, but the oily slick of troll juice had stuck me granite like to the floor. My lips mouthed a silent 'help me' scream, which sighed away breath-like on a frosty day, and disappeared.

I slowly turned my eyes to the ceiling. The little pits sprung springs of streaming saltiness that overflowed and traced the contours of the mask-free face which was not mine. Yet still I felt their warmth against the unfamiliar icy cheeks. I wasn't crying or sobbing, I just lay there, perfectly, deathly, still. The springs kept spilling out the sorrow I no longer had room for. And I no longer had control.

I lay and waited to die. Not long now I thought. Not long now. Not long now.

Hushed whispers in the corridor.

My mother and the doctor appeared in a halo of light in the doorway.

The doctor on a Sunday! Now I knew things were serious, very serious indeed.

He checked me over as I lay.

"I can't get up. I can't move. I feel like I'm about to die. I can't go to school. What am I going to do? What am I going to do?"

The words tumbled, jumbled in the torrent of tears.

"I can't go on, this is the end. I've got nothing left."
Complete despair.

The doctor sat beside me. He reached for his battered, brown leather bag, the kind that all doctors have, reassuring, strong, and unbreakable. Doctors' can cure everything from their magic bags. They have the whole world in there. The cure for lumps and bumps and aches and breaks, all crammed into a crumpled case. No wonder they bulged. Magicians in the healing field.

"You are very ill," he spoke softly as if not to disturb the fading light that calmly caressed the room. "You should have been put on antidepressants a long time ago, and you must see a counsellor. I'll write you a sick note so that the worry of returning to work will not bother you for the time being, and I don't think you will be well enough to go to work for a while yet. You must go and see your own doctor tomorrow to sort these things out and I will tell him I've seen you. Don't worry about anything, your mum and dad are here to look after you, and if you need me just phone... Look after yourself."

He got up, picked up his magic bag, and disappeared in a puff into the halo of light.

I lay in the darkness.

CHAPTER SEVEN

I stood at the gates of the house. I must have walked past it thousands of times, but I never knew what went on behind the secure stone walls which protected it from prying eyes. From the way it looked I had always assumed it was a care home for the elderly. Large and grey it loomed with white, bright windows and a cosy conservatory, warm and welcoming. The wandering wisteria had wrapped its way around the walls and hung like a comfortable overcoat. It looked quite nice for a mental hospital. I crunched my way up the drive, tummy full of dancing butterflies. What if they think I'm a fraud, what if they think I'm okay, what if they say nothing's wrong? What will I do? What will I do?

How could anyone see inside my head and see that it was broken? You can see a plaster cast on a leg or on an arm or on a foot – something for sympathy, something to sign in recognition of the hurt. But bandaging a brain was a lot more difficult. If you can't see something hurting or bruised or battered or broken then it isn't. It just isn't. If you can't see it, there's nothing wrong, so everything must be okay. That's what people thought. I was sure of that.

I had at last admitted, and given in to the fact, that I was ill. I didn't have an alternative. It had completely smashed everything that I had become, everything that was me, and all of the layers of protection and barriers I had built castle-like around myself. Everything was gone and I was left with someone new yet oddly familiar, someone I hadn't met for a long, long time. It was a very awkward feeling, a little like when you meet someone at a party that you haven't seen for years and you just can't place them. You hesitantly shake their hand and rack your brain trying desperately to remember who they are, where you've seen them before, and just what their name is.

I looked at the stranger in the mirror. I looked deep into her eyes and I could see someone sad, confused and unwell, yet I thought I remembered knowing her once upon a time. I was ashamed. How on earth could my life have come to this? How could I have become so very ill?

But with the admission that I was indeed ill, and that it wasn't all in my imagination, came an indescribable and enormous amount of relief. I was finally given permission to stop plugging the leaks and cracks and holes in the dam, and let the pressure smash everything to bits, and I let it wash away the rot and debris in my life in one uncontrollable, powerful wave.

So here I stood, wrecked, washed up, and dripping. Not knowing where I was or who I was or where I was going, but I was ready. Ready to begin resting and rebuilding the dam, inch by inch, pebble by pebble, in a way that was right for me. In a way, that would stand the test of time and was strong and unbreakable. In a way that would enable me to swim in the cool, tranquil waters of happiness, contentment, and peace, once I had finished building it.

This would be my first stumbling step. This would be where it would all begin. So I pushed through the door with my heart in my throat, and held on tightly to the first smooth glistening pebble in my hand.

The room where I waited was sparsely decorated and slightly grey, with shabby but comfortable chairs to sit in and spill out from. My eyes were drawn to the view of the rambling garden, beautifully bushy with sprinklings of coloured flowers, their buds now beginning to open. They looked so sweet sitting there I could almost smell their fragrance drifting through the air. And as I sat I watched the dull drizzle that had now begun to draw stripes in the dust on the window, behind which I trembled in the little grey room.

A man, who I assumed was the doctor, and a lady, who was the psychiatric nurse, entered the room and introduced themselves. They looked quite young, in their forties, and I was very relieved they wore no white coats. They smiled with their clipboards and said they were there to assess me to see if they thought I would actually benefit from their help. They asked me what I thought I might need to resolve in my life, what I might like to talk about. My palms were sweating as I wrung my hands tightly together trying hard to think of all of the things I mustn't forget to say. This was my chance, my one and only chance – my chance to have someone there to listen to me, to be there, to help. I really didn't want to mess this up and fail. Fail as I always seemed to do, and which always left me coping on my own, once again. I had to get this right. My eyes fixed firmly in my lap, and I began quietly, mumbly stumbling, to reel off the list of events and feelings and things that had brought me here, to this place, in this mess, to the mental health unit. When I had finished my quiet request for a little help to resolve the pile of life that had squashed me flat, I tentatively raised my soggy eyes to see if I had passed or failed or been rumbled as a fake or a fraud or somebody normal. Tissue pressed to nose I searched their faces desperately looking for a clue. Their eyes matched mine.

"I see many people here Rachael, who come for one problem or situation that they need help with, which they need to resolve or to talk about. You have come to me with at least ten of these problems all at once. I really don't know how you have kept going for this long; you should have been here months ago. You are amazingly strong to have kept going; most people would have given up a long time ago. We have a lot to talk about so I definitely want to see you as soon as possible next week," the kind-faced lady said. The doctor nodded his head in agreement.

I left the hospital feeling a little fuzzy and dazed. I thought that maybe I wasn't such a failure after all. Then I thought I was a failure. Then I wasn't sure.

CHAPTER EIGHT

From the moment my eyes first cracked open in the morning, until I crawled between the covers at night, I felt only two things: overwhelming exhaustion and fear – great, big, brimming, buckets of fear. Fear of everything, absolutely everything. Everything I used to do, everywhere I used to go, everybody in my life, terrified me. The only place I felt safe, the only place I felt a little bit secure, was at my childhood home with my parents. Quasimodo had the bells, I had my mother. And when I caught a flicker of light in the darkness and dared to dream, it was the only place in the world I felt things, one day, a long way away, might just be all right.

Each day I crowbarred myself from between the sheets. Not an easy task, as all I wanted to do was to twist myself into a tiny knot between the covers and stay there all day, forever and ever and ever. But I knew from somewhere a long way away, in my strange and mixed up world, that this was not the answer. A distant whisper from a misty memory occasionally found the right frequency and signalled a disjointed direction.

It told me I had to establish a daily routine to try and bring some order to the chaos. Everything was upside down and back to front, smashed, broken and unrecognisably scary. So I figured if I brought some sort of ordered, controlled pattern to the day, things might get a little easier, a little better. Control over an out of control, chaotic existence. That's what I needed, so that's what I tried to do in my own crazy way, from the bottom of the dank and dirty hole I had fallen deeply into, breaking everything except my bones.

So I summoned all of my strength and got up to face a world I did not like and did not want to know. I forced myself to shower. A pointless exercise it seemed. How can you wash off the black disgusting dirt when it was all on the inside? But I went through the motions every day, then put on my black joggers and black jumper for my black life. I didn't bother with make-up any more. What was the point, my secret was out, the mask was broken, and I was ugly on the inside and ugly on the outside, and it just seemed like a complete and utter waste of time. Make-up makes you look good and feel good and I wasn't either, so I didn't bother. By the time I had done this I was exhausted, so I would crawl back into bed for a couple of hours sleep, then try again to get up and face the world.

I knew in my heart I couldn't hide in the house, my protective prison, forever. If I did I might as well give up the fight now, glide to the gallows and dangle dead. So every afternoon I forced myself, no matter how difficult it seemed or how terrified I was, to go outside and walk. Even if it was only for five minutes, I knew I had to push myself into being in the same world as the human race. The race I felt I no longer belonged to, and feared I would never be part of again.

Slowly, stiffly, I would shuffle; Shoulders sagging and eyes staring and staring at the concrete pavement, making sure as it rippled and bucked beneath my feet that I wouldn't fall flat on my face, or down a crack, and have to start all over again. My heart would be pounding so viciously that it felt like it had taken over the whole of my insides and was about to explode my ribcage out and spear the passers by. Pumping and pounding it squeezed and crushed my lungs, so that after each step I took I gasped desperately for air. It had rung my insides so tightly that I leaked through every pore, which helped to drench my flaming face. Each time I went out I prayed to the Godless sky that I wouldn't see anyone, and that they wouldn't see me. I wanted to be the invisible woman. If I don't look at them they might not see me, I thought. They might not look into my staring, glaring, empty eyes and see that I am officially insane. I was sure as I toed along the invisible tightrope I used to guide me in a straight line, that everyone could see what I was, how useless, and dirty, and frightened I was, now that the mask had gone. No wonder they stared and stared at the naked troll. If I saw someone coming towards me I would change direction, take a turning, or cross over the road so as not to let them get too close. I didn't want anyone to see me the way that I was, and I didn't want to frighten anyone with the freak show that was me. Sometimes I got trapped. Sometimes I couldn't change direction, turn a corner, or cross over the road, and I would be terrified. Heart stopping, screaming, terrified. As they came closer and closer I was convinced they were going to stare and stare and point and point and rumble me and shout, "Hey look everyone, this girl's a nutter! She should be locked up! She shouldn't be allowed out here with us 'normal' people! Look at her!!" And they would point and point and laugh and laugh and I would crumple crushed, and die of embarrassed humiliation. As they got closer my heart would pound louder and louder and faster and faster and my head would swim and switch my focus off as I gasped and gasped for breath. As they got closer, my head would scream and scream until I couldn't move or think or feel and my brain could not and would not function. And the person would pass me by and not notice me writhing on the floor in pain and fear and terror. Then the feelings would sluice away leaving me a quivering puddle of wreckage. Every day I undertook my quest hoping that it might, one day, just one day, become a little less scary. And that I wouldn't have to go back to bed afterwards trembling, tired, and as always, terrified.

But I would not, and could not, give in.

It wasn't just strangers I didn't want to see, I didn't want to see anyone. Not friends, not family, not anyone. I stopped phoning everyone, and I would not take the calls of anyone that rang. I couldn't go through the lying pantomime of,

"How are you?"

"I'm fine."

I was not fine. I couldn't lie any more. But I just didn't have the strength or the courage to explain the truth. I didn't want anyone knowing what had happened, and what the truth was, that I was mad, and that I had failed. I withdrew into my shell and sealed it up water tight against the tempestuous sea that tumbled and battered outside.

One day I remember a friend coming to bring me some flowers. She knocked and knocked on the door. I didn't want her to see me; I didn't want her telling anyone what I was really like, how bad I was and how bad I looked. I lay on the bedroom floor in my grubby, red dressing gown. I was convinced she could see me hiding there, on the floor, like a slug, with her X-ray vision. I was sure she could see me and she was laughing and she couldn't wait to tell everyone how pathetically stupid I was. I was sure she was going to somehow unlock the door and come on in, and point and laugh and laugh and laugh at me huddled in a heap on the floor. Of course she didn't, she just left the beautiful bouquet, which I didn't deserve, on the steps of the porch, and then went away.

When I was really, really sure she had gone I poked my hand out through the crack in the door and retrieved the present of petals and perfume.

'With much love from all of us,' it said. I cried.

CHAPTER NINE

I sat, curled up in the chair, in the little grey room with Sylvia, my psychiatric nurse. She was forty-something with short pepper-flecked brown hair, a stylishly earthy sense of dress, and she always wore strings of wooden beads. I often thought that maybe they were worry beads. But her face was calm, serene, open and kind, with soft but penetrating cool blue eyes.

I felt very safe with her and, in an odd kind of way, loved.

I knew today would be the day I would have to begin to turn myself inside out and empty everything that was me onto the floor into a huge, steaming, jumbled pile of mess, and have a really good look, whether I liked it or not. And I suspected not. I was determined to dredge the dump and throw out all of my life's rubbish, then I would keep the good bits, after I had examined them closely, pop them back into their boxes, and I would then file them away in my memory chest. I was going to have to be totally honest, and totally ruthless, no matter how painful things were, or how embarrassed I was, I knew I had to do it. I was being given the opportunity to have a sparkling, bright, white new chance of starting my life afresh, and to do this I had to get rid of the ghosts, the debris, the rot and the cancer that had eaten darkly away at me, deep inside, for the whole of my life. To do it I had to be honest with myself and my feelings, and I had to begin now. I had nowhere left to hide from myself.

Today we were going to talk about two things. The first was about me, my general background and a brief look at the things that I had done in my life. The second thing we were going to talk about was my childhood, a kind of an overview of the way things were before I entered into the complicated world of adulthood.

What on earth could I say about me? I thought hard as it wasn't easy. I wasn't sure what she wanted to hear, and I didn't want to say anything wrong as I might not get another chance to begin sorting my life out, and to make things right. So I tried my best and began to whisperingly and cautiously unload myself.

Well, I was twenty-seven years old with blondish hair and green eyes. My father was an environmental officer, my mother was a journalist and I loved them both very much. I was brought up in a small town, in a middle-class environment with my younger brother. I had a 'normal' upbringing and a 'normal' academic background. I did GCSE's, A' Levels and a B.Ed (Hons) Degree. Once I left college I worked as a teacher in an infant department in a private school. I was a kind, caring, intelligent person who had loved animals, writing, art and painting, but now I had no interest in anything. That was all I could think of to describe me and my life. Everything just felt flat and dead and all of the things about myself that I used to believe to be true I was no longer sure about. I didn't enjoy anything any more, and I didn't know where I was going or what I wanted. I wasn't sure if the things I thought I liked I actually liked, or the things I thought I disliked I actually disliked. I just didn't know. Everything was topsy-turvy, so I left the description of the sad stranger I no longer knew at that.

Now for my childhood: I closed my eyes tightly and tried to think back as far as I could to my first memories; tried to think if there were things that had happened which might have shaped me into the broken jumble of mess that I was now.

From a very early age I had always felt a dark cloud of sadness hanging around somewhere near, never quite going away and leaving me to be a happy carefree child. I don't know why it was there or how it got there, but it was always there making me feel bad, making me feel like I wasn't good enough and like I didn't fit in. I always felt different to everyone else, I always wanted to be accepted, and in my mind I never quite was.

When I was four I first started school and I loved it. I loved learning and I loved my friends and teacher. I had started a term early for some reason, which meant when my friends moved into the next year I was left behind to start the year with children of my own age. From then on I felt like I didn't belong, like I had been left behind because I wasn't good enough to move on.

I was always bigger than everyone else, taller than everyone else and developed a lot faster than everyone else. I always wanted to be sweeter and smaller and blonder and more fashionable, but was always a big black blob. I always wanted to be cute and naughty and fussed over like my brother, but I always had to be the responsible older sister. Very serious. My parents had always shown me so much love and kindness, but I always felt that I wasn't the one they really wanted. My mum had lost her baby daughter, the one she really wanted, then she had me, the replacement, then she had my brother, the golden child. That's how it seemed to me since I was small. Now I realise I was very wrong to feel like that, but that was the way it was, that was the way I felt, and I told no-one. Feeling this way had left me with a huge desire to be accepted, to do the right thing, to please my parents, to make them proud of me and love me and forgive me for being the replacement. I carried on looking for approval and acceptance for the rest of my life.

We moved to Australia when I was eleven. I hated it. I never fitted in there at all. The sunshine, the golden sands and the warm blue seas were beautiful. School was not. They were all Australian in my class and academically far more advanced. I had gone from being one of the oldest in my class back home, to one of the youngest in the class in Australia. Different academic years you see. They were all bronzed and athletic. I was fat and blobby and the only one in the class to be already wearing a bra. My God! The humiliation! They all swam in their pools, in the sea and anywhere they could like a shawl of glistening, gliding fish. I bobbed about like a lump of dumpy driftwood. They mocked me. They mocked me for lots of things, but mostly for being a "bloody Pom." I only had two friends in my class. One was called Kylie, a strapping Kiwi who really didn't care at all what people said. She also didn't fit in, being a Kiwi and living in a caravan meant that people weren't that interested in her either. Well she didn't have a pool did she? My other friend, called Carly, was, and I can't put this kindly, the class 'smelly kid'. She was ginger, painfully thin, always smelt and dribbled when she spoke. She had trouble writing and reading and she thought I was great, a friend just for her. I felt really sorry for her; she was taunted worse than I was. I didn't care if the other kids were horrible to me because I was friends with her. She had offered me friendship, which was more than they had done, and that was fine by me. I dreaded going to school each day. I found the work hard, I found the taunting hard, I found the isolation hard, and to make it worse I knew my brother was having just as much of a rotten time in his class as I was. He kept running out of his lessons and going home, so my parents had enough trouble with him without my unhappiness being another burden for them. So I didn't tell them how I felt. I knew they had lots and lots of other problems without mine, I wasn't sure what they were but I knew they were there.

My mum cried a lot, and my dad lost stones of weight and turned into a grey skeleton. He still couldn't find a job.

And then my grandfather died; a heart attack two weeks before he was due to come and join us with my grandmother. I remember mum sitting us on the beach, wrapped up in jumpers, as the sky raced past in shades of grey and the sea, deep green, swished foam onto the sand.

"I want you to be very brave," she said through glassy eyes. "I've got something very sad to tell you... Grampy Bill has died." The ground opened up and I fell in. I didn't stop crying for days – days and days and days.

My grandmother still came, but with her she brought her mother, my great grandmother, Nanny Joan. And I knew everything was going to be okay, Nanny Joan was taking charge.

"Rice pudding is the answer," said Nanny Joan, and we believed her. The sun was blazing in and it must have been 90 degrees, but we all sat around the table and did as we were told. My father, stick thin with sunken eyes, my mother and grandmother puffy faced and red eyed, and my brother and I sat sadly, quiet and scared. Nanny Joan dished out huge steaming platefuls of sweet home made rice pudding from a pot the size of a dustbin. Even the stray tabby Tiddles had his own bowlful beside us. It was the most deliciously fantastic thing in the whole world, and I glowed from head to toe. I felt better. Everyone smiled. I knew everything would be okay.

We came home soon after.

We arrived home in the Summer just as my final year in junior school would have been coming to an end. I went to the end-of-school disco, the highlight in every child's school year. I was so excited to be seeing all of my friends again, and slotting back into our little class foursome, as we had been very close. We had done everything together, shared everything with each other, and when we were all together I felt like I belonged. I felt like I fitted in and was actually part of a very special group of friends. But when I arrived at the school gates my friends rushed out to see me, but instead of there being three of them there was four. I had been replaced, and things were never quite the same with five.

I became close to just one of them, Nicky, through my senior school years. We were inseparable and did everything together and shared everything together. The 'overripe twins' they used to call us. We never quite fitted into any of the social groups, not the trendies or the hard nuts or the swots, so we were friends with everyone, but no-one in particular. I think that's how we survived senior school unscathed. That's where I learned to be a social chameleon. Then one day, when we were about fifteen, Nicky got a boyfriend and that was the end of that. She spent all of her time with him and he controlled her. She wasn't allowed to call me or see me or go out with me. He saw me as a threat to their relationship for some reason that I never fathomed out, and all contact was cut. I felt like I had been abandoned, bereaved. I had lost the closest person to me, my confidant, my partner in crime, my friend. I couldn't understand what I had done to deserve this or what had happened, and I was stunned and I was angry – angry that she never had the courage to stand up to him and say "Hey! I will see Rachael if I want to!" Or maybe she just didn't want to. She had been my very best friend since I was five years old. I was numb, glum and very, very lonely. I had been rejected yet again.

I knew what rejection felt like, I had been rejected before.

There had always been friction between my parents and my father's parents. It had gone on under and over the surface for years. One day it came to an explosive head and dad and mum decided the best thing was that they didn't see them any more; too much pain. Sometimes these things happen. They told my grandmother and grandfather that they could ring us or come and take us out any time they liked, as they didn't want to deny us our grandparents, and they didn't want to deny them their grandchildren. They only had to call, but they never did. I could never work out what I had done wrong. I could never understand why they hated me so much that they didn't want to see me ever again. I never did know the answer. I still don't.

When I was deserted by Nicky I really needed someone to talk to but found that everyone scurried away into their little holes, away from Rachael when she actually needed them for a change. I was angry. I had always been there for everyone, absolutely everyone.

And now they had disappeared. I was an emotional dumping ground for everyone throughout my teenage years. People came to me and talked and talked, and cried and cried until I had helped them unravel their life, picked them up, dusted them off and pointed them off in the right direction again. People came to me with every type of trauma life had to offer. I had helped gay people, abused people, raped people, bereaved people, people on drugs, people who drank, people who decided that dying would be the better option, and held the hand of my friend, alone with her abortion. People felt they trusted me, could confide in me and I would know all of the answers. I was a fountain of knowledge for trauma and pain. Mostly I did understand, sometimes I didn't, but I would always help. The sad thing was that once I had helped someone they would suddenly keep their distance. It upset me at first, but then I realised that they were embarrassed because I knew their deepest darkest secrets, so they felt exposed and very, very vulnerable. Silly really, I never thought any less of any of the people who came to me once they had told me their troubles. Sometimes I thought about turning people away when they came to me so that there didn't have to be any of that embarrassed awkwardness afterwards, but I never did. I cared too much and wouldn't see anyone upset or in pain or frightened, so I just put up with the consequences of 'being there' and carried the load alone.

I talked about all of these things with Sylvia. I wasn't sure whether the things that I had spoken about were relevant or not as they seemed like a jumbled bag of nonsense. Many children had a childhood a million times worse than mine, mine was almost idyllic, so how could I sit there and say that these things had upset and affected me. I felt quite guilty. But as I thought hard about this I realised that if I felt I had to tell her about these things then they were painful, and they did affect me and they did matter. They mattered to me. And as I sat and listened to myself and the things that I said, I realised that at a very young age I had totally lost my confidence, so that everything that came after in my life was built on a crumbling foundation. I began to realise that all of the things that upset me and haunted me from my childhood were made worse by the drip that was fed to me by the darkness. Whatever the darkness fed me I believed it to be my reality. I began to realise that I had built the whole of my life on the illusions of the dark angel and maybe, just maybe, not on the truth. The darkness was my gospel. 'You're fat, you're ugly, no-one likes you, everyone laughs at you behind your back, you're useless, useless, useless,' my dark angel would grin, and I believed her. Somehow I had to find a way of silencing her for good…Forever. Maybe then the silent snowy one would be able to squeeze from the tiny box that I had held her prisoner in for as long as I could remember, and see if she could still use her tiny, silvery, singing voice before the darkness silenced her for good.

CHAPTER TEN

Lots and lots of people get ill with lots and lots of different illnesses: some are curable, some are not, some are on the inside, and some are on the outside. Some people never even know that they're ill and that something dark and deadly is crawling, scraping, and quietly nibbling away inside of them until it's too late. They've drawn the short straw of life. Bad luck. One thing I knew was that all of these ailments, diseases and disasters had all been written about at some time or another; a book for everything, telling you all about the pain and the pus and the rashes and the incurable aches. The symptoms, the illnesses, the cures and the consequences all rolled up and bound together by the smiling face of a beardie weirdie doctor who claimed to know all about it, or so he says. "Read all about it! Read all about it! Roll up, roll up, and have a look at all of the things you hope you'll never get!" Everyone likes to know about these things, delving with morbid fascination, wanting to know a little bit about this, wanting to know a little bit about that. You just can't help yourselves can you? Have to just take a little peek, like rubbernecking at a road accident. It's human nature you know, you don't have to be embarrassed.

Well I was embarrassed, standing in the library amongst these books. There was shelf after shelf of books of all shapes and sizes and colours, telling you about anything and everything you wanted to know. It had taken an enormous amount of courage to come to the library on my own, where people might see me and stop and stare and point. But I decided I had to go if I wanted to try to make myself better. I had to go and find myself some books on the illness that I had. If the doctor was indeed telling me the truth, and what I had was a real illness, then there must be a book on it somewhere. There were books on every other illness so I couldn't see why not.

I stood wide-eyed and mesmerised in the medical section, desperately hoping no-one would see me. I slowly inspected every title in that section, looking for something that might be relevant. Would it be under 'Mental Illness'? Would it be under 'Depression'? Would it be there at all? I just didn't know. I couldn't bring myself to ask one of the librarians to help me as talking to strangers was far too traumatic for me, and anyway I was far too embarrassed. How could I possibly ask the librarian for the type of book I was looking for? I didn't want her to look over the top of her horn-rimmed glasses in a knowing and patronising way and tut under her breath at me. So I carried out the laborious search on my own. Eventually I found quite a few books on depression, amongst books on phobias, anxieties, self-esteem enhancing and others associated with the mind and all of its complicated facets. I was really surprised to see quite how many books there were on the subject, and to me that said two things. The first was that what I had was actually a recognised illness as there were books on it in the library. The second was that if there were quite a few books on the subject then it must be quite popular, which either meant quite a few people had depression and wanted to find out about it, or there were a hell of a lot of voyeurs out there who liked finding out about other people's misfortunes. Either way I realised that more people knew about this illness than I had realised. I chose two books about depression that looked quite interesting, although they did seem very clinical and medical. I couldn't find any at all with a 'human' view, so they would have to do. I also chose a book on how to develop high self-esteem, and my goodness I needed to develop that. I wasn't sure if it would help or not but I figured that I had to start somewhere, and I needed all the help I could get. Then I went to the art section. I decided to try and rekindle the interest that I once had in art and beautiful things, to remind myself of what I used to like and who I used to be. So I chose a book about colour. Start at the beginning, I thought, at the basics. I wanted to try and help myself to remember that the whole world was full of brilliant colours and beauty. I wanted to help myself begin to be inspired, and think and feel again. To try to help see colours flickering again in my life and all around me, instead of everything being varying shades of black. Black feelings, black thoughts, black life. I wanted to see Piccassos and Monets and Klees, not 'Black cat in soot' and 'Drizzle on concrete'. My gallery had become very limited. No wonder I didn't want to visit it any more.

I was pleased with my little haul as I went up to the counter to check the books out. I could feel my cheeks begin to flush and my temples begin to throb at both the thought of having to speak to a stranger, and the fact that she would see my selection of books and know that I was slightly loopy. I didn't want her feeling worried or on edge at having to deal with me, and I certainly didn't want to make her feel as uncomfortable as I was feeling. I piled my books upon the desk with the book of colours on the top of the pile, shielding my dirty dark secrets from the outside world. I wanted it to mask the other books in my collection for as long as possible, so that I could put off the embarrassment of what I was, and so it would disguise the contents of the books that I had underneath it. I felt like a dirty old man hiding his porno mag inside his copy of 'Fisherman's Weekly' so that no-one would realise what he had and what he was really like. The librarian treated me surprisingly kindly and courteously, and strangely for the first time in a long while I felt a little bit like a functioning human being. It was an odd feeling as it flashed past me, but I caught the feeling briefly, for one moment in time, and I kind of liked it. I felt like I had accomplished something that day. So I placed another pebble in the pile.

Trying to read the books was another matter though, as I had the concentration span of a flea in every activity I tried to undertake. I could sit in front of the television for an hour and I wouldn't be able to tell you what had happened in the programme I had just been watching, sometimes I couldn't even remember which programme I had watched. And sometimes I just fell asleep right there in the chair, curled into a little foetal ball, a little full stop. The concentration it took to try and focus on the television totally wore me out; I found it really hard. It was the same with conversations. My attention span was so poor that someone could be talking to me and I couldn't tell you a word that they had said and I certainly couldn't reply in a sensible and coherent way. I would get really close to their face and stare with manic concentration deep into their eyes, or watch their lips, hoping that if I watched them really, really closely that I might be able to understand what it was that they were saying. Sometimes it seemed to me that they were speaking Russian or Latin or Hebrew for the amount of sense it made. And I would be willing myself to try and remember just one single thing from the conversation that would prove to everyone, and myself, that I had one little cell functioning correctly in the memory department. The frightening thing was that often I couldn't even remember seeing the person that I had spoken to, let alone remember what we had spoken about. Most of the time someone had to remind me who I had seen and what had been said. Sometimes when people recalled this to me I would vaguely remember a splattering of the conversation and sometimes when people reminded me I would deny categorically that I had even seen that person, let alone chatted with them. Either way, once I had been engaged in a conversation for more that about five minutes, the intense concentration I had needed to participate in it drained me of every drop of energy I had, and left me crawling droopy eyed into bed for an energy regaining nap.

Everything had become such an intense effort and my short-term memory was also appalling. I would forget what I was doing, where I had put things, what I needed to buy when I got to the shops and almost everything anyone asked me to do. I used to get so frustrated and annoyed and angry with myself. It would really upset me that I was so terribly useless. I wanted to help my mum so much, as she had been so kind, that when I forgot to do the things that she asked me I would cry with frustration at my pathetic stupidity. I remember one day she rang me up from work to ask me to take some sausages out of the freezer for our tea. By the time I had put the receiver down and walked into the kitchen I had completely forgotten what I had gone in there for, and had completely forgotten that I had even had a phone call from my mother. It was hopeless. Luckily everyone who was close to me, especially my mum, knew how difficult things were and would just laugh it off, even though I was sure they must have been tearing their hair out. They never showed me they were angry, and we would all laugh at my hopelessness. It became a standing joke. It was good to laugh, it kind of defused upsetting, frustrating and difficult situations in a good and positive way, and I was very grateful for that. There was never any pressure or pep talks, and I was never told what I should be doing or that I should "pull myself together." That would have possibly been the most damaging and destructive thing that anyone could possibly have done. Living the nightmare I was living was difficult and traumatic enough without the pressure of people telling you that you should 'sort yourself out' and 'there are people in the world a lot worse off than you'. I knew that, I knew that, I knew that! Saying things like that would have only increased the tremendous guilt that I was already feeling and have put me under unbearable pressure to get better a lot quicker than I was indeed able to. The people around me were brilliant. There was never any pressure, no dates at which I would have to be better by, no-one minded if I slept all day, or if I didn't speak to anyone, or if I curled catlike into a ball in the corner of the room to protect myself from the world outside. No-one minded, no-one commented, they only cared and made normal my abnormal behaviour. The way they behaved was an integral part of my healing process and I was, and still am, eternally grateful to them.

I sat with the book about depression in front of me and opened it at the first page. Another mountain for me to climb. I squinted and began to concentrate on the trail of words that meandered out before me, into the distance and beyond. I read sentence after sentence, trying desperately to hold my wandering brain together in one place long enough to be able to absorb the information I was drinking in through a blocked straw. Sometimes I was able to read a whole page and was able to retain and remember it. Sometimes I would have to re-read a page, two, or three, or four times, in order for me to absorb what it was that I had read. Sometimes I couldn't get to the end of the sentence without forgetting what it had been about. Reading was certainly an uphill battle with lead boots and a lead brain. As always I would have to sleep afterwards to recuperate all of the energy that had been sucked out of me whilst concentrating on the reading. Sometimes I even fell asleep with the book on my lap, or on my face, and would wake up confused and forgetful and not know where I was let alone where I had got to in the book, and I'd have to start all over again. It was really hard work. But, through determination and painful perseverance I began to read word after word, line after line, and chapter after chapter, and forced and forced and forced myself to try and remember the things that I had read. And at last, after a couple of weeks of struggling, sleeping, phone calls from the library reminding me I had forgotten to renew the books (surprise, surprise!), and brain straining I finally managed to finish one of the books. I was very pleased with myself. A pebble pile of three. It had been really, really difficult but I had done it, and what I had read amazed and astounded me. It was as though the whole book on depression had been written about me. Special Forces on 'Mission Impossible' had crawled into my ear, surveyed and sampled the seething swamp, and reported back to base with their findings. A nasty, dangerous job, but somebody had to do it. And there it was, laid out before me, in black and white for all to see. It told me about the physical, psychological and emotional effects that depression has on a person. It told me about the symptoms you might see and the behavioural changes you might have. And it told me that all of the things I was experiencing and had experienced were 'normal'. Me normal. Now that was a revelation! It also told me that one day, after a lot of healing, and healing took time, that I would get better. In my heart I wasn't quite sure if this was true, but it was written by a doctor, so it must be true, I'd just have to keep hoping and trying. The book also said that you would go up and down in peaks and troughs, highs and lows, highs and lows until you got better. The lows would be very low with tiny blips of high, then back to low. Then the highs would last a tiny bit longer between the long lows. Then the highs would get longer and longer and the lows would get shorter and shorter, and eventually you would find yourself somewhere in the middle and would feel a whole lot better. I surely hoped so. It also said not to give up or feel frightened when the lows kept coming back, as this was natural and it would seesaw, seesaw, until you were balanced again. It was so reassuring to realise that there were some people out there who actually seemed to know about, and understand, what I had been, and what I was, going through. This was a proper illness, and I was a textbook case, a shining example, a specimen. A specimen in a little glass jar, choking on my own filthy air, being prodded and poked and stared at until one day I would be released and I would be free. Free to float away and fly and fly and fly way up into the clear, bright, sunshiny sky. Until I could smile and shine and soar, and until my heart would burst with happiness. Until it burst my ribcage right out, spearing and popping the rainbow bubbles all around me and showered glistening glitter everywhere. I held on to this thought, kissed and caressed it and put it in my pocket, so that I could get it out and have a peek, whenever I liked, whenever I needed reminding, at my little sparkly dream. My dream was a long, long way away from being my reality, but at last I was beginning to crawl.

CHAPTER ELEVEN

I looked at Sylvia's kind warm face as she encouraged me to talk about the main painful splinter from my childhood, the one that had burrowed its way deep inside me and stayed there, rotting my heart and rotting into other areas of my life. I could see her kindness quietly spilling out as she patiently sat in the little grey room waiting for me to spill myself out, whenever I was ready. It was as if we had all the time in the world, and nothing else mattered except me and what I was about to tell her. I lowered my eyes and stared at the hands that were clasped tightly in my cross-legged lap. I couldn't look at her, as I was embarrassed and ashamed about what had happened. It was all my fault.

I had known Dean since I was eight, and he was eleven, and I had always thought the world of him. We used to both get the coach on a Saturday morning and go to the music school for orchestra practice. I used to play the violin very badly, and he used to play the drums, both at the same place, but in different orchestras. We got on so, so well and would always sit by each other on the coach and share our sweets that we had bought in the tuck shop at break time. He was such a witty, charming and bright boy, and he would fool around, as most boys do, and I would laugh and laugh and feel quite privileged that he was my special friend. Sometimes he'd play the coach seats with his drumsticks, he was really good, and I would be in awe and brim with happiness.

I remember the day I told him I was going to Australia. I saw him walking up the road, he'd gone to the local senior school two years before and he looked really smart and handsome in his bottle-green uniform. His long dark wavy hair bobbed as he ran towards me, we hadn't seen each other for a while, and he beamed from ear to ear. When I told him the news his pale green eyes welled up with tears that burst the bank and flooded out over his face full of freckles. We both cried as we walked away in opposite directions. I thought that it would be the last time I would ever see him and I was heartbroken. He was too, judging by the overwhelming reaction he had when I had told him the news. Some people may say that I was far too young to feel true love, that it just wasn't possible. But that's what I felt. I knew I loved him, I had done since the age of eight, and every time I saw him my life would light up like the most magnificent Christmas tree, and I would smile for days.

When I went to senior school I saw Dean nearly every day, which was wonderful. We'd always have a laugh and a joke and chatted about lots of different things, but we never got too close, as it just wasn't 'cool' for him to be hanging around with a younger girl like me. Then one summer's day, when I was fourteen and he was seventeen, a most marvellous and magnificent thing happened, Dean asked me out. I was so happy I thought I might just pop as I got myself ready. I put on my favourite tight, bright, yellow top and skirt and my white winkle-pickers, the ones with the cotton wool jammed into the ends to stop the toes curling up into a goblinesque style. I carefully put on my make up and tied back my long curly hair with a yellow ribbon. I looked in the mirror and thought I looked fantastic. I had been waiting for this day since the age of eight and now, at long last, my dream had finally come true.

As I was only fourteen the places that we could go to on a date were a little limited, so when he said we were going to his friend's house I was only slightly disappointed. At least we were going to be able to spend time together on our own, and this made me feel sparklingly special.

I stood at the door with Nicky, butterflies skipping in my tummy with excitement. She was going out with Dean's friend so it made a cosy little foursome, and life just couldn't get any better. We all laughed and chatted and had a lovely time, then Nicky and Matthew decided to go to the shops to get some crisps and coke. Dean and I stayed and watched television. Dean held my hand and little tingles tickled my fingers and electricity sparkled and danced between us, and then he kissed me. My whole world lit up. I bubbled inside like smiley sherbet and, fizzing, floated on the ceiling.

Suddenly something changed. I don't know what and I don't know why, but it changed. The sweet sherberty kisses became rancid and rasping and made their way over my face like satanic slug slime. Vice-like fear grasped my insides and held them tight. Something was wrong. I wasn't sure what it was but a deep primeval sense was screechy screaming its alarm from deep within, firing instructions. 'Fight, flight, freeze; Fight, flight, freeze. Quickly, choose one, Choose One, CHOOSE ONE!'

I looked deep, deep into Dean's eyes as his grip became tighter and the putrid rasping rougher, and I saw a raging black soul, unrecognisable, intense, evil, penetrating back from the eyes of a stranger.

"No-one can see you, no-one can hear you, no-one will know and no-one will believe you," he spat at me, "I want to hurt you like you've hurt me."

I didn't understand what he was talking about. I hadn't done anything wrong. Yet I was being cruelly punished for what ever it was I had done inside his sick, sick mind.

He tore at my clothes with one hand like a salivating raging beast, stretching and yanking and tearing, and undid his clothes in a frantic frenzy. His other arm nailed me down across my throat, so that I couldn't breathe, and I gasped fishlike for breath. Both of my arms had been pinned tightly behind me, underneath his and my weight, and I had been pushed so hard back into the sofa that the springs dug deeply into my back through the cheap-smelling foam.

I couldn't feel the pain. My brain had made its choice, and I had stiffened and was frozen, with eyes as big as fear and disbelief-filled saucers. I couldn't shout, I couldn't scream, I couldn't move, as the sickness spread through every inch of my body and chilling ice spread its spiky fingers through my stomach, slowly down each limb, pierced and sliced my heart, and froze my brain in terrified inaction. Confusion, fear, disbelief and shock drove one stake into each limb, and there lamb-like I lay, corpse-cold and sick-filled. And the coldness that spread through me was black and rancid and poisoned me on the inside, it would never go away.

The searing pain in my head, in my heart, and in my body smashed me into a thousand pieces but at that moment I couldn't feel it, for the icy sick had frozen it out. This was the day that changed my life forever.

A noise at the back door broke the voodoo spell, and as he stopped I pushed him with one enormous shove that burst up from the soles of my feet, through my body and into my arms, gathering tidal wave force as it went, and I knocked him off. His face was horror-filled as he realised they were back, and I ran and ran to the bathroom and slamming the door, I locked myself in. My body violently shook and shook and tears washed down my face in torrents, and I retched and retched and retched to relieve the poisonous black sick that was drowning me on the inside. When the sea of sick subsided I looked at my smudgy shipwrecked self, through my tears, in the mirror. I tried to see if it was me, if it was real or if it was a dangerous, deadly dream. But it was painfully real, reflecting back at me in glorious Technicolor, reflecting the painful shameful truth. I wiped away the black slick of make-up that had slithered down my face and tried to flat down my hair, as my ribbon and slides had been lost in the struggle-less struggle. I tried to soak away the little maps of blood that had found their way onto my skirt with little soggy pieces of tissue that stuck to them like flags. X marks the spot, it all happened here. I dabbed and soaked and cried and tried desperately to compose myself before going downstairs and escaping. I didn't know what to say, and I didn't know what to do, so I spun around in the whirlwind inside my head and landed in the kitchen, instead of Kansas, with Nicky and Matthew.

"Have you two had a row? Dean's gone home," they laughed. I began to try to tell them what had happened but they both laughed and said 'don't be so silly' and that 'he's a really lovely bloke' and 'he wouldn't do a thing like that' and 'it must have been some sort of misunderstanding'. I shut my mouth and wobbled home. I didn't tell anyone else what had happened. I was so completely shocked that I wasn't sure how I was supposed to react. It wasn't a dirty stranger in a dark alley, it was someone I knew and trusted and loved. I didn't know whether to shout and scream and rant and rave, or curl up quietly licking my wounds, or go and report it as something serious. I just didn't know what to do as I was so, so upset and confused. So I sat in the eye of the tumbling turmoil and hoped it would all blow away. I thought about telling my parents but didn't want them to have to feel the pain that I had felt. It was best that he only shattered my life, not that of everyone around me too, and I didn't want them saying that I had been stupid and I had done something wrong. I was so ashamed and embarrassed and guilty. It was all my fault. I was sure everyone would think it was my fault. If only I hadn't gone, if only I could have seen what he was really like, if only I had shouted and screamed and kicked and fought then none of this would have happened. I had cared for him, loved him, respected him, and trusted him with all of my heart, and he had betrayed it all and smashed my world apart. He had been perfect in my eyes, so what happened must have been my fault. Or so I thought.

As I sat huddled, cradled in the chair telling Sylvia of the pain I had locked away inside for thirteen years, it felt like yesterday. I trembled and cried and felt the coldness spread deep, deep inside. The wound had been gashed open again, but it needed to be as it had never healed properly in the first place. It was a festering, rotting, gaping gash, and at last maybe now I was ready to fill it with antiseptic and sew it right up.

My whole life changed after that. He had used me as an object, a mucky feeling-less, worthless object. I felt so dirty and disgusting and ashamed on the inside, it began to show on the out side. I threw all of the bright clothes that I had away and replaced them with varying shades of black. My make-up went from powder blues and pearly pinks to raven black and blood red. And my long curly locks were shaved into skinhead spikes. I screamed 'don't come close,' so no-one did. It was my defence, my barrier, my warning. If I scared people away I couldn't be betrayed and hurt and soiled and smashed again. I trusted no-one.

I didn't feel like I deserved to be loved, as I was dirty and contaminated and ugly, on the inside and on the outside. I was worthless and useless and it was all my fault. I was so deeply ashamed and embarrassed that guilt gnawed away at me blackly every day. My clothes were black, my face was black, my bedroom was black, my music was black, and inside the blackness blinded me. I coped and coped and buried it away deeply in a Dean shaped coffin. I was strong, I could cope; I told no-one.

A year later my friend Susan came quietly to consult the 'oracle' with tears welling silently as she spoke. She didn't know where to go; she didn't know what to do. So trembling she came to me. She told me a story of a boy that she had met in a drunken haze at a party. They had mistakenly had sex and afterwards, realising her mistake, she tried to leave. The lovely boy that she had met locked the bedroom door and suddenly turned into an unrecognisable raging monster. He beat her and threw her around the room as she tried to struggle away and leave, then he brutally raped her. She showed me the bruises. I felt her pain.

How would anyone believe her when she had already had consenting sex with him, I found it hard to take in myself. But the tears, the pain in her eyes, and the bruises were a shining testimony.

"Is it anyone I know?" I asked gently.

"I'm not sure if you know him, his name's Dean."

My stomach shot into my mouth and filled me with an old familiar icy black sickness. Suddenly I was in the room with her. I could smell what she smelt, I could see what she saw, I could feel what she felt. I was her and she was me and I shook with her. This I could not cope with. This I could not do on my own. I needed to get help for her, and for this I needed someone else. How could I possibly advise her when I couldn't even help myself.

I went to our head of year at school to get his help and advice for her, paving the way, as she was too ashamed to go to see him. As her story tumbled out mine tumbled too. And when I finished the things that I had to tell him, I searched his face for some kind of reaction. But none came, as his face was frozen in open-mouthed shock. When he finally composed himself and regained the appropriate air of authority, he promised to help Susan. My pain wasn't important I kept telling him; I just needed him to help her. He smiled kindly and his face softened as he gently said,

"I think you need to talk to somebody too." So I thought about it a little, and decided that maybe it was time I did.

I sat nervously in the Victorian room at social services with its high ceilings and comfy chairs. The squinty, bespectacled, middle-aged counsellor sat with me, with uptight hair and uptight clothes, a lemon-sucked face, and comfortable shoes. She was totally grey in every respect.

I will never forget her opening line, the worst thing in the world she could possibly have said. It all went downhill after that.

"I've been told that you have a problem with your father," she said over the top of her spectacles, through her pinched lips. It was her way of getting me to open up and say "Oh no, it was something quite different!" and spill the beans on what had really happened. A forest fire of anger and resentment burnt through me. How the hell dare she insinuate anything, ever, about my father! He was the most wonderful, kind and caring man I had ever met. He was my hero. My anger surged through me to the point where I wanted to smash her to bits, but I held it inside. I was good at that. I corrected her monumental mistake, hissing through gritted teeth. My shell had clamped closed and I knew I just couldn't talk to someone as stupid as she clearly was. I gave her a short and sharp version of what had happened, as at the age of fifteen I didn't have the courage to walk out there and then and point out helpfully the error of her ways. She spoke to me in the most patronising way and insinuated that maybe I had 'led him on' or that I had 'misunderstood him'. Is she for real? I thought. I even thought that maybe I was being filmed for one of those wind-up TV programmes, but figured that no-one could possibly be that cruel. The final straw came when she told me in her nursery teacher's voice that next time she would bring two dolls with her, so that I could show her what he had done. I was fifteen years old, not bloody five! I raged out of the room like an exploding firecracker, I was so, so angry. She dragged my father into the dirt, insinuated it was all inside my head and spoke to me like I was five years old. I had trusted her with the most traumatic and secret part of my life, the part that I had never told anyone about, and this was what I got. I vowed I would never, never, never see her again as she was the most vile person I could imagine, and I decided I was better off coping in my own lonely way. I sent her a letter to say that I was never coming back, and I never did.

It took me seven years to let a man get close to me again. Even then it was sometimes very difficult. I had to feel completely loved, and completely trust someone, before I could let them anywhere near me. And as soon as the love and the trust began to waver and fade in a relationship, as it always did as I had a knack of picking the 'wrong kind of man', things would become difficult for me. A wrong look, a wrong touch, a wrong word, from someone where the love and trust was fading, brought me vivid horrific flashbacks. Not of faces, but of feelings. They would trigger an icy sickness in my stomach that would spread through the whole of my body and send me silently screaming and crying and retching and retching and retching to the bathroom, where no-one could see me, and no-one could see the depth of the pain. My whole body would tremble and tremble and it would take a while for the pain to subside and the chill to go away. But I coped. I always coped. I had to.

Sylvia and I talked and talked and talked about what had happened and how I felt, and I began very slowly to see the truth. It didn't get rid of the blackness, it didn't get rid of the pain, but it began to slowly dissolve some of the guilt. And when the guilt had gone, then maybe, just maybe, the pain and the darkness would go too. I really, really hoped so. It was not my fault. I had done nothing wrong. I had reacted in a way that any woman might have, and I had only been a child. I had only been a child, dealing with an adult's problem, on my own. Now I was not on my own. Now I was being taken seriously. Now I was being made to see the truth about what had happened. It was not my fault. It was not my fault. It was not my fault. I was not dirty, I was not contaminated, I was not a bad person. I had to learn that there were loving and kind and trustworthy men out there, although I had never found one, and that they were not all vile. It would take a very long time for this to sink in, but at last the black sick's stubborn stain was beginning to be scraped away. I was making a start. I had a lot to think about.

I held a pebble, smooth and cool, in my hand and turned it over and over between my fingers, wondering whether or not I should add it to the pile. I hadn't achieved anything, but I had made a start, so I put it on the pile and smiled.

Each time I came out from one of the counselling sessions I felt absolutely and totally, physically, mentally and emotionally shattered. I always felt like I'd just been slugging twelve sweaty rounds with the hammer-fisted heavyweight champion of the world. I could hardly walk and certainly couldn't string a sentence together, but my mum would be there waiting and smiling with open arms and a huge hug. She'd always take me for a glass of cool white wine and a plate of crispy curly fries after my session as a little reward, even if it wasn't lunchtime. She knew how shatteringly painful it was each time I went, but she was always there, always smiling, always strong. I knew that each prick of pain I felt she felt too. I knew it was hard for her, so very hard. She felt so guilty. 'If only I'd done things differently, if only I'd stepped in to stop this all happening, if only I'd have known about all of the troubles I could have helped,' she would say. She had done nothing wrong. She had done everything right, but she still felt guilty. I tried hard to reassure her but I could see the hurt in her eyes. She had nothing to feel bad about. She would sometimes ask me after a session if I had talked about her, if she had done something wrong, if she had brought me up badly, if it was all her fault. But it wasn't. It was my fault. I was the one who had let myself tumble into this black hole, and I was the one who had to climb out of it, by myself. She could certainly not do any more than she was doing. She was great even though she didn't really truly understand. To me it didn't matter that she didn't understand, as long as she was there.

CHAPTER TWELVE

Mum and I stood at the entrance to the supermarket. She took me once a week; my weekly dip into real life. I absolutely hated going to the shops, big ones, small ones, the butcher's, the baker's, the candlestick maker's, it really didn't matter, I hated them all. It didn't matter what I was going in to get, or how long I was in there for, I detested every second of it. And I could never go into a shop alone, someone always had to be there, be with me, holding my hand. I hated it, but had to do it, had to try, had to make an effort to make myself better.

The large mouth of the supermarket grinned and gaped and encouraged us to be swallowed up into Consumerland by the bright white light that shot out like a tractor beam guiding us into the mother ship. Taking a huge deep breath, and screwing the lid more tightly on to my maniacally wriggling nerves, I stepped into the light.

Inside the craft was a different world. Everything seemed so bright and white it peeled my eyes through squinting slits. The brightness shone from everywhere, bouncing in every direction, off every thing. An icy silvery blue aura hung mist-like in the air, giving everything an unnerving and unnatural florescent hue. There were no dark corners, nowhere to hide. I was illuminated on the stage from every angle, so I would hang my head hoping no-one would see me, hoping the curtain would fall before everyone could laugh at my dire performance.

I always pushed the squeaky, wayward trolley around after my mother, but to my horror, and sometimes amusement, the trolley always took me on its own little tour, to exactly where it wanted to go. Each time I hung on tightly to it so that I had a base, a crutch, something to keep me from swooning and collapsing under the crushingly bright lights. And it always helped to hold me upright as I withered from the boring eyes of the greys. They seemed to wander in mechanical pointlessness, pushing and shoving at intervals to break the predictable monotony and frustration of the shopping and of their lives. They seemed angry and irritated to me, but their faces were expressionless, featureless, eroded by the tide of life. I could tell they were looking and waiting to find something, anything for them to look down on and mock to make themselves feel better about their own sad lives. I tried hard not to make any eye contact at all, and would stare at the front of my trolley making sure it didn't swing me into the back of someone's ankles and cause a row I couldn't cope with. I could feel their eyes staring and deeply penetrating me as I tried to mingle, trying to look normal with my trolley full of this and that, I knew not what. All of the time, I tried to keep my face expressionless, so that I would blend in and not show anyone how terrified I was. I would trundle wonkily past the plump piles of purple plums, and towers of teetering tins following my mother as best I could. She always chose the food and the things that we needed, as I didn't have an opinion. I didn't have an opinion on anything. My decision-making skills had long since deserted me so it was easier for others to make my decisions for me. Even if I was asked if I would like a chocolate biscuit the answer would be yes...no...I don't know...I'm not sure, what should the answer be? It was hopeless. If anyone asked me to make a decision about anything I would tremble, flush hot and cold, and stutter, unable to get my brain to supply me with a simple answer. It was like having a scratched record that would get stuck in repetitive indecision until someone lifted up the arm and placed it down again giving me an answer. I couldn't decide what I wanted, what I preferred, what I liked, what I didn't, and I never knew what I wanted to do or where I wanted to go. The only thing I always knew was when I wanted to sleep, and that was only because my brain and body demanded it.

I hated the pulsating blinding lights and the mumm, numm, mumm of the fridges and the freezers and the lights, lights, lights. And the bumbling hum of the swarming grey wasps as they squished and squashed their way down each aisle, bumping each other out of the way. And sometimes they would bump me or faintly touch me as they flew by, and I would fight the rising urge to be sick as they had made me dirty and had contaminated me with their uninvited touch. Even getting too close and sharing their air made me feel sick inside. The thought of breathing in the same stench-filled air that had been inside their lungs horrified me. It would make me tremble with rage, how dare they touch me with their grubby hands, how dare they blow their own foul air into my lungs, how dare they look at me with their angry miserable faces. Why couldn't they just leave me alone? Always looking, always staring, always judging, they had no right, but still they terrified me. My head would thump and thud and the aisles would become smaller and smaller and the people would become bigger and bigger and I would find I couldn't move and I couldn't see and I couldn't breathe and I was trapped, drowning in the murmuring swarming mass. Heart racing, head pounding, eyes swimming, and a rising swell of sickness and twisted cold nerves inside my stomach. It was terrifying. Claustrophobic, consumed, trapped. I had to force myself to breathe in big gulpfulls of air as my lungs were crushed and frozen with fear, and concentrate like mad on not screaming and run, run, running away from the fluorescent, glowing, pulsating mass. Sometimes when it really got just too much I would hold mum's hand, like I was five, just for the reassurance that she was there and everything was okay. At least I was there; at least I was trying; at least I didn't give up and concede defeat. Sometimes I would be very brave and go off and look at something in the shop on my own and say I would meet mum five minutes later in a certain place. This really helped, except for the time mum was a little late meeting me and I searched and searched and looked and looked and my body began to overflow with terror at the thought of losing my mother and being trapped inside a shop, on my own. I stood there terrified not knowing which way to turn or what on earth I was going to do, and then I saw her, blissfully unaware of my consuming panic, and when I saw her I cried and cried and cried. I was so relieved, the panic washed away, and through the tears I began to laugh and laugh at how ridiculous I was and how ridiculous I looked, but I really didn't care. I just saw the humorous image of one of the shop assistants holding my hand and leading me to the Tannoy system to make an announcement for a 'lost mummy', and the lost little girl only being twenty seven years of age. Sometimes I laughed at the way I was as I felt ridiculous, but I couldn't help the way I was, I just had to do my best to get better. No matter how stupid I felt or how stupid I looked I really didn't care any more. That's why I always made a special effort when it came to standing in the queue to unload the trolley and pay with my mother. Everything inside me screamed 'run away, run away, run away,' run away from the lights, run away from the people, run away from the ever increasing fear as I stood and waited and waited and waited. It was horrible. But when I trundled, wobbly zig-zagging out of the shining mouth of the ship, I smiled and felt triumphant. I had survived, I had not made a fool of myself, I had not collapsed, and I don't think that anyone had noticed or had even cared about me looking a little odd and out of sorts. The shops were always an ordeal, but at least I battled with them, lance in hand and trusty wayward steed in front. And as I unpacked the shopping, I'd unpack the glistening pebble at the bottom of the plastic bag, and I'd smile.

I stood at the big wrought iron gates of the school looking at the rusty brown pebble before me. A huge pebble to put in the pile with the others, but I wasn't sure if I could lift it. I wasn't sure if I was strong enough. The building was large, red brick and overpowering, and stood well within its rolling established grounds. I was wearing my smartest black trouser suit and had my large black leather portfolio under one arm. I had been told about the job in the primary school by another teaching friend who worked in the school. It was an excellent school and an excellent job; an opportunity not to be missed. Whatever possessed me to think that I could cope with an interview I do not know. All I could think was that I knew I could never return to the school I was teaching in, too many memories, too much pain, and I was too embarrassed to face all of the parents and the staff there. I didn't want to be judged by people who didn't know the truth and didn't understand. The parents were difficult enough when you were one hundred percent and on top of the world, always quick to jump, quick to complain, quick to moan, such hard work. Even for a conscientious, creative and caring teacher like I had been, they were still, at times, unbearable, creating an awful amount of unnecessary pressure. I thought a change, a fresh start, something new, was perhaps what I needed; a job to look forward to doing in September, rather than dread. The dread, I felt, was holding me back and not letting me get better as quickly as I should. So I had gathered all of my courage together and applied for the job. And my goodness, I had got an interview! I was elated. I was not as useless as I thought I was. I thought even if I got there and sat and cried or fell over, at least they had thought that I had been good enough to interview, and I was chuffed. I spent ages that morning putting on makeup to liven up the new face that I had discovered when the mask had broken into tiny pieces and fallen off. It felt quite odd. I was enhancing rather than disguising, and it was all completely new to me. Once I had livened up my complexion with peachy blusher, brightened my eyes with pearly eye shadow, and painted a rosy happy smile onto my lips, I looked in the mirror and was pleased with the results. Today, at least, I could pass for a member of the human race.

I had asked my father to take me to the interview as I knew the forty-five minute drive to get there would have wiped me out. I just couldn't drive that far as I knew that after about fifteen minutes of driving my concentration would lapse dangerously and my eyes would begin to unfocus themselves. Then soon I would begin to feel myself slithering down the driving seat, and would be held upright only by the tight grey safety belt. So dad took me and dropped me right at the entrance to the school. So there I stood, waiting to go through the porthole to another world, another dimension where I was a normal human, able to cope – a number one employment candidate. After spinning in the phone box, I stepped through the gates, and entered the school as 'Rachael - Super Teacher'. I strode down the corridor, which was entirely decked in dark, carved, wood panels, like a luxurious manor house, and my shoes click-clacked behind me, signalling my arrival. I felt like a completely different person.

I was shown around the school by the head of the infant department, Mrs Jones, a short lady with a green tweed suit and a greying bun tied back tight and practical behind her head, with nit-avoiding precision. She twitched her tortoiseshell glasses up and down on the end of her nose as she spoke, and the gold chain of the glasses jingled as she told me of the school and the rooms and the children and the great expectations. I smiled and chatted and soaked up the school, trying to remember everything. The schooly, woody, disinfectanty children smell filled my nose. A murmur of industrious, excited, chit-chat floated on the air from each classroom as we passed. Each room sounded different. Each room bulged with a different type of excited enthusiasm. And each wall was filled with colourful, creative, painted cats and castles and elephants and rockets and flowers and smiles and they all shone out gleefully from the children's displays of their treasured artwork. I had always admired enviously young children's creativity. They painted things not only as they saw them, but they painted how they felt about those things. It was always amazing to me how detailed and expressive a young child's work was, and how they were never given enough credit for the talents that they had. People never seemed to realise that if you gave children the skills of mixing the colours that they wanted, and brushes big enough for them to handle, but small enough to allow them to show the detail that they wanted, then they would produce brilliant things. Move over Piccasso! Most people would give small children three different ready mixed colours, big stubby brushes, make them paint on a vertical easel, and wonder why they didn't produce pictures of any quality. Could you with those tools? It would pain me to see the frustration on their faces when they stood back to admire their work and would stare at it with dissatisfied teary eyes, as the paint had dribbled its way down the sheet of poor quality paper and down their sleeves, and the beautiful flowers had drooped and covered themselves in rivers of streaky mud.

I was smiling, I was passionate – I felt alive.

As we walked around and chatted I could feel Mrs Jones warming to me, and we exchanged views and ideas and questions, then we came to the door of Year One. This was where I was to read a storybook I had brought with me to the class of five and six year olds. I was terrified inside but I thought to myself, 'you have done this thousands of times before, this is not difficult, you can do it, you can do it, you can do it - if you can't do something as simple as this then you might as well give up teaching right now.' I peered through the glass window of the door. Year One. This was it. We knocked and pushed open the door. It felt comfortable, yet odd, as I hadn't been in a classroom for months and months. I hadn't been anywhere for months and months. The floor was covered in an industrial burgundy carpet, which had been slightly worn by over-enthusiastic scuffy five year olds. From each wall shone rainbows of paintings and collages. There were carefully mounted stories written in 'very best' handwriting, and posters and pictures of letters and colours and numbers and all sorts of informative things. There were the children's names in large bold print, each one on a coloured list to show who was in each working group, and a lovely chart with everyone's name on it, and by each name was a glittering row of stars to show who had done some excellent work. The chart was battered and dog-eared by enthusiastic star recipients, sticking on their star vigorously as they burst with pride at the recognition of their hard work. Sometimes I wished adults had such things – recognition of enthusiasm and hard work and achievement in life.

The children were huddled in groups all sitting on their little orange chairs doing very important business. Some had counters and maths books and number lines and quizzical expressions. Some were reconstructing chopped up sentences extracted from their reading books so that they made sense, then writing them neatly into their books with their favourite pencils. Some were standing with bright red aprons on, at tables covered in newspaper. They each had a stern look of concentration on their face as they tried to figure out how to attach the toilet roll to the cereal packet in order to make a highly sophisticated intergalactic communication device. If only the glue would stick this on and not glue the box to the table and stick my fingers together in such an annoying way, their faces said. As I walked in their bright eyes all turned in my direction, and a ripple of tiny whispers began. They tried hard to conceal their excitement at someone new coming in to read them a story. The teacher interrupted what they were now not doing, and assembled them onto the blue carpet in the reading corner. I sat down in the comfy brown corduroy chair with yellowy, wooden, varnish-chipped arms, and got out my storybook. They wriggled a little in anticipation as I introduced myself.

"Aren't you all sitting beautifully," I fibbed in a voice of calm authority. "Now let me see who is sitting the most beautifully." It never failed. The carpet full of wriggly bottoms now sat neatly, wide-eyed and concentrating, all eager to be picked as the 'best'. I said that I couldn't possibly pick the best ones as they were all so very good, and they all beamed, we had connected, and I began the story. I loved telling stories to little children as they became so completely absorbed and transported into the story, and I found it such fun doing the voices of the characters and reading with expression and meaning. The expressions on their faces were wonderful and they changed with each twist and turn of the tale. Fear, excitement, sadness, fun, happiness and awe all showed in their faces as the story was read, and they all strained intently to look at the colourful pictures that I showed them at the end of each page. I had chosen an exciting, interesting, fun and colourful story, which I was sure would capture their imaginations as it had done before with other children. It went down very well, they loved it, and I brimmed with happiness and confidence.

After I had spent some time with the class I was taken by Mrs Jones across the rose garden and lawn to the main building at the centre of the school, and was led into an echoey, stone-floored entrance hall. We wound up and up and up a never-ending stone staircase, which grandly swept around all four walls of the hall. It seemed to go up forever. As we went up, on each level, there was a large window displaying yet another expanse of view, always showing a different aspect of the vast school grounds and buildings. Eventually we reached the Gods at the top of the tower, and in an enormous square wooden clad room, which oozed opulence, sat the Headmistress at her solid wooden desk, on a huge green leather chair. She eyed me up and down, and smiling beckoned me to take a seat at the desk with her. She had beautiful strong features, thick wavy naturally blond hair that framed her face like an old style movie star, and she wore a classic lilac suit. Her voice was strong and authoritative, yet soft with a hint of a lilting welsh accent. She was mesmerising. We talked freely for a while, and I showed her proudly some of the work I had done with other children and some of the things that we had achieved, and I felt on top of the world. At the end of the interview she shook my hand warmly yet firmly, and thanked me for coming and showing her these interesting things. As I walked out of the large iron gates I felt an enormous sponge fill my head, my legs buckled beneath me, and I headed in completely the wrong direction to the pub where I was supposed to be meeting my grandmother for a lift home.

I was elated, but completely and utterly shattered. It had taken every last ounce of energy to do what I had done, and I felt pleased. Even if I didn't get the job I still felt elated as I placed the rusty brown pebble I had picked up at the gates onto the small but slowly growing pile.

Mrs Jones rang me the next day to say that she had really enjoyed meeting me and she had enjoyed looking at my work, but unfortunately I hadn't got the job. I wasn't entirely surprised as I was sure that there were better candidates than me, I just hoped and prayed that this was the reason that I didn't get the job. I hoped it wasn't the fact that I had let myself down badly, and not realised that I had indeed come across as not being able to cope, and not quite normal. I really hoped I hadn't let myself down, I really, really hoped. One thing I did realise from this experience was that the more I thought about returning to St Mary's in September, the more it filled me with dread, and the more I was paralysed with fear. Having an interview had knocked me sideways and I had spent the rest of that day and a lot of the next sleeping, and when I was awake my head was full of mashed potato. I was at last beginning to acknowledge the fact that I wouldn't be able to cope with full time teaching by September, the healing process was taking an enormous amount of time, and progress was very, very slow. I thought about it long and hard and realised that by September I realistically wouldn't be able to cope with the pressures that teaching brought with it, and I would never have the energy to last the long and hard working days. I would miss the children, I would miss the close friends I had made with the staff, I would miss the beautiful school and I would miss the pride I felt at being a teacher, but I knew in my heart of hearts I couldn't go back. I didn't want to keep them hanging on indefinitely as to when and whether I was going to go back. And I knew if I let them know now they could advertise straight away and get a teacher that was the cream of the crop. So with tear-filled eyes I walked to the little red post box with the full stop in my hand, and with a little hesitation and a few more tears, I posted the letter away. As it disappeared into the darkness with a hollow plop I felt a tremendous sense of loss, but at the same time a tremendous sense of freedom, and I also felt a little of the weight lift off of my sagging shoulders.

The next day, I received a letter with the bright blue and yellow school crest upon the front. I was totally amazed that they could have received my letter and replied to it so quickly. I ripped it open to see the reply and as I unfolded the neatly typed letter my face dropped with horror as I read what was before me. It wasn't a letter accepting my resignation. It was a letter from the headmistress, which I guess must have crossed with mine in the post. I couldn't believe my eyes as I read how she said she didn't know that I was applying for other jobs, was very surprised to see that I had managed to go for an interview whilst I was supposed to be off sick, and requested that I go in to school and 'explain myself' to her. I was stunned and horrified. She already knew I was applying for other jobs, as even if I could get better in time to go back in September, I certainly couldn't survive on the under-scale wages at St Mary's, the cause of some of my financial problems, and I had already told her all of that. So why was she lying and hassling me like this? And what on earth was I supposed to do? Was I supposed to just stand by and let myself fall deeper into the hole, or try to do something about it? And why on earth should I have to go in to see her and 'explain myself'? I felt like I was being reprimanded like a child. And I was not a child. I felt wave after wave of fear and sickness sweep over me, and my whole body shook, I was terrified. She didn't think I was ill, she thought I was shamming; she thought I was going behind her back; she thought I was a liar, liar, liar. And she must have thought the doctor was a downright liar too, filling in those sickness forms with gay abandon when there was nothing wrong with me. What was I supposed to do? Was I not allowed to try? Was I not allowed to do the things that might just help a little to get me better? Was I supposed to sit in a darkened room and let my life disappear in a swirling swish down the plughole and do nothing about it? Was I not allowed to go out, to try and do the things that I found so hard, in order to do something, to do anything in order to make myself better? I shook and shook and cried, terrified she thought I was a fraud, terrified she would expect me to go back to school straight away, terrified if I did go back that I would expire and die as I had nearly done before. What did she want, what did she want, what did she want? I became more and more traumatised and hysterical as I walked around and around in circles, shaking violently and gibbering to myself, not knowing what to do, what to do, what to do. I phoned the doctor and went straight in.   An emergency. An emergency as I had become hysterical, I was frightening myself, and the devilish, demonic, bad, black thoughts had raced back in, trying desperately to make me do something I might not live to regret.

I felt sorry for the doctor afterwards, having an inconsolable sobbing wreck quaking and raving for forty minutes, and all the time waving the evidence – the letter, the thoughtless bloody letter. The poor man finally managed to calm me a little and through the blanket of hysteria I remember him saying I had done the right thing by trying to do something positive about the situation. I was not going to be made to go back to work, they couldn't make me do that, and I wouldn't be able to cope. I was still very ill, and I wouldn't be well enough to even entertain the thought of going back to work for a while. And if she had any problem with my illness, and if she wanted any conformation of the truth, then he would speak to her and, in no uncertain terms, put her in the picture, put her straight. He told me I was doing well to try and do some of the things I found so, so difficult and this was all part of my recovery. And most importantly, it was not my fault – I had done nothing wrong. Then he checked me over and increased my medication. I had already had my medication changed once as it was not working, and now the new medication was being increased. Making sure I was on the correct magical marvellous medicine was not as straightforward as I had first thought. Maybe now I would begin to get somewhere with it and actually feel it helping.

I was deflated, exhausted, and disheartened. I had tried so hard and had had it all violently kicked back in my face, blinding me, making me stumble, and making me lose my wobbly balance. And tumbling, I lost my grip and slid and skidded backwards towards the familiar grinning gaping black pit, knocking loose rocks and debris as I fell, which bounced and scattered into the screaming blackness beneath me. I slid and grabbed and slid and grabbed and managed to grasp some tufts with bleeding fingers and broken nails and stopped myself from sliding further. I am not going down there again, I hissed through gritted teeth and salt smeared eyes, I am NOT going down there again.

CHAPTER THIRTEEN

I sat and stared out of the window at the metamorphic plump puffs of grey and white that marched determinedly across the sky, billowing and bulging into different shapes as they went. I watched intently as little bits of bright blue sky peeked through and waved. Little glimpses of hope. They reflected and waved back at themselves from the shimmering puddles, and the glistening grass shook itself, refreshed. At least it had stopped raining. My gaze returned to Sylvia's warm and smiling face, and I began to tell her about the relationships that I had had up until I met Guy. There weren't many, but the ones that I did have came with huge and insurmountable problems.

I had met Phil when I was twenty-one and he was twenty-six. He was about six foot tall, blond, bald and bulbous, and he had chubby cheeks that would flush and pulsate with blood when he became enraged. We had met in a pub, he was completely drunk, and I should have known then how things would be. Not long after we had met I foolishly thought that I was in love with him. He was the first person who had shown an interest in me, someone who I felt I could trust, and he was the first boyfriend that I had had since Dean. I trusted him quite quickly for some reason, I'm not sure why, perhaps it was because he seemed so genuine and different from all of the shagnasties that I had met at college and had kept at arms length. They had all seen me as 'one of the lads' at college, which was great for drinking beer and watching rugby, but not so great for being taken seriously as girlfriend potential. And I still wore my 'keep away' disguise of total black, and red hedgehog hair, which worked as was intended, and left me on my own. I often wanted to show them me, the real me, a feminine lady, loving, kind and vulnerable, but never felt I could. I didn't want to be laughed at, so I carried on being a boy.

Phil though was different, because he actually wanted a relationship. He seemed like a gentleman, he had a good job in navigation in the Navy and I was very proud of him. In the beginning it was roses, meals and romance, before he went off for his next stretch at sea, and I was totally smitten. We wrote to each other all of the time and he would ring whenever he could. It was awfully exciting and romantic, and it wasn't a problem that he was away for a lot of the time, as I was away at college and was always very busy. Things seemed to be going well until I saw a little flash of something I really didn't like when we went to his sister's eighteenth birthday party. We arrived at the local rugby club where the party was being held, and I was filled with a certain sense of excitement. Whenever I had been to parties before it had always been with friends or family, but never with a boyfriend, and I felt very happy and very proud. We walked into the shabby, noisy, smoke-filled bar, which was heaving with loud, sweaty, already drunk people all pushing and shoving to be served at the understaffed bar. Puddles of beer soaked their way into the tattered beer mats, and tin foil trays of infected peanuts and fag ash sat in spilled sophistication on the bar, as we waited for a flat pint of beer in a plastic beaker, and a warm glass of vile cheap wine which made your eyes cross and your lips shrink and stick onto your teeth. As soon as we had got a drink Phil began some stupid, macho, drinking ritual with his ex-army, barrelesque bald father, and both of his jack-the-lad younger brothers. My stomach began to clench as he drank more and more and began to get drunker and drunker, and I became more and more worried and more and more lonely. It was like he had something to prove, something to live down to, just wanted to be 'one of the lads'. Then Phil disappeared, I couldn't find him anywhere. Suddenly his vile tempered, vile mouthed sister came bursting in through the saloon doors, on spiky red vinyl stilettos with her bleached candyfloss hair floating out like a yellow storm cloud around her head. She was in floods of tears, Phil and one of his brothers were fighting outside on the rugby pitch. I was flung to the side as his lurching father rampaged outside to sort things out. I'm not sure how things were resolved but all three of them came back in dishevelled and grassy, covered in a dazzling array of cuts and bruises, and his father held a ruby stained hanky to his nose. Phil had hit him too. I was really shocked and really frightened. I couldn't believe he had got so drunk, and was so full of anger that he would fight with his own brother, and punch his dad. They all seemed quite jolly after their little escapade, a jolly jape for the boys. And his short and spiky mother rolled her eyes and pursed her lips, but smiled because she was proud of 'her boys'. I had begun to sober up quickly and started to become fearful as to what the rest of the night would bring, and how on earth I was going to get home safely. I asked him gently if maybe he had had enough to drink now, but he leered and spat that he hadn't had enough and who the hell was I to tell him what to do. As the evening went on I lost him again, then spotted him just outside the bar surrounded by a group of jostling, shouting people, all pushing and shoving, and sharing the peanuts as they watched the show. As I got closer I could see that he had picked a fight with a local nutter who had a reputation for being a psychopath and a very handy fighter. Sweat and beer and fists were flying everywhere as the bouncers struggled to prize the scrapping animals apart. His face was full of rage and covered with beer and blood as I dragged him out of the door, away from danger and repercussions, and headed for home. I was supposed to be having a lovely time, but I wasn't, I was looking after a drunken, disgusting, irrational animal. I was upset and angry and embarrassed. How could he have done this at his sister's eighteenth birthday party, and when he was supposed to be looking after me? It was too awful to contemplate. I wasn't sure if he was the man I wanted to be with after all, but he won me over as he always did, with his flowers and presents and sober charm. I had seen something that day that I really didn't like, but I buried it away, hoped it wouldn't happen again, and tried desperately to ignore it.

Things carried on and on and on. Every time he got drunk and humiliated himself, and me, I ignored it and pretended it didn't happen. Every time he got drunk and abusive towards me I ignored it and pretended it didn't happen. Every time he got drunk and had a fight with friends, with strangers, with his brothers, and with his uncle at another family party, I ignored it and pretended it didn't happen. If I ignored it and buried it deep, deep inside then maybe it wasn't happening, maybe it wasn't real. When he was sober and caring and loving it didn't seem real, it was easy to pretend these things didn't happen, but they did.

I would be full to the brim with fear and dread if I knew we were going to go anywhere where there would be alcohol. He knew he had a problem, and would promise me faithfully every time we went out that he would only have one or two pints and that he would behave himself. But he never did. As we walked into a pub and that familiar malty, hoppy smell hit my nose, I would begin to feel scared and sick, and as I saw him put the pint glass to his lips my heart would sink. And each sip that he supped would change him, mouthful after mouthful after mouthful. And each and every mouthful would make him louder and louder and more and more angry and obnoxious, it was embarrassing and it was frightening. I should have finished the relationship as soon as I had realised, I should have walked away, but I didn't. I didn't because I was scared. Scared of being on my own, scared that this was my only chance at a relationship, and scared because I didn't think that anyone else could ever possibly want me. I was surprised that Phil had wanted to be with me, my self-esteem was so, so low. I had put my faith and trust in him, the first man since Dean, so I had to stay with him. I convinced myself I had to make it work, as this, I thought, was my one and only chance. So I carried on burying the fears that I had and tried hard to make Phil face up to his problem. When he was sober he had a problem, when he was drunk he didn't have a problem, apparently. So on and on we went.

One day, out of the blue, Phil asked me to marry him. I was delighted. I never thought that anyone would ever be interested enough to even go out with me, let alone actually want to marry me. I accepted. I didn't feel like I had a choice. If I didn't say yes then the relationship would be over, and I didn't want it to be over because I felt like no-one else would ever want me. I also foolishly thought that he might change, he might just see the problem that he had, and fix it, and everything would be okay. I was so naive. Things didn't get better though, they began to quietly spiral down and down, getting worse and worse. His drinking became heavier, his anger intensified, and his abuse got worse. And as the drink slowly took hold, he would become more and more angry, more and more abusive, louder and louder, and angrier and angrier. I was convinced that one day he would actually explode from his seething anger and lash out and hit me. I was sure it was only a matter of time as I was already his easy outlet, his emotional punch-bag. When we went out I would watch him, filled with worry and pain, as he got drunker and drunker and drunker. Then he'd begin pushing and shoving and swearing and shouting, and his face would twist and contort in blood vessel bursting anger. Until he was so angry and he'd blown up so far, that once we got home the final glass of whiskey would be the pin prick in the balloon which would fire him off around the room and deflate him into a shrivelled pile of passed out pukiness. But still I persevered.

He decided to leave the navy and go to college to do a science degree. He had had enough of being away at sea and needed a change. I thought a change of environment would do him good. He got a place at the college that I was just leaving, which I found odd. It was as if he wanted a piece of me, and a piece of my life. Like he was jealous of what I had had, and wanted the same, wanted better, wanted to show me he could do it too. I couldn't understand what he was trying to prove; he didn't need to prove anything to me at all.

Then he began to turn on me even when he hadn't been drinking. Every time I achieved something in my life he would sneer, find fault and downright ruin everything I was ever excited about or proud of. When I got my degree results we ended up having a raging row when I rang up to tell him. He was supposed to be coming over to go out and celebrate with me and my friends, all of whom were deliriously happy and excited with all of their results, but he turned it into a showdown. I had to drive ninety miles to be with him, he said, or nothing. I chose nothing. I wanted to celebrate with him and my friends and I was determined I was not going to let him spoil the most exciting day of my life, and the last time I was going to go out with the friends that I had been with every day for the past four years. I was not going to let him spoil it this time, no way. He didn't even say congratulations, or that he was proud of me, he had decided he was going to spoil it and that was that. We didn't speak for days.

When I got my first temporary full-time teaching job, at what I thought was the most amazing private school, I was so excited that I thought I might just burst with pride. He became angry.

"You might not like it, it might be horrible, they might not renew your contract," he said blackly. He never said well done, or that he was pleased for me. And they did renew my contract. He was angry about that too. I couldn't understand it. Then one day I began to realise that he was jealous of me. Jealous of me, the things I had achieved that he had not, the things I had that he did not, the friends I had that he did not. It was crazy – crazy, crazy, crazy. If he achieved something or had something good or did something good, I would be so happy for him and proud and excited. I thought that's how it should be when you're in love, when you're partners, when you're engaged. You should share each other's joys and triumphs. He obviously had other ideas.

He was living away at college by now, and when I returned from college I had moved back in with my parents. I felt it was now time to move out and live on my own, so I began looking for somewhere to live. I found a nice house on an estate, which on paper I could afford, and bought it with the intention of having a lodger to stay with me. There was no way I could afford to live on my own until Phil left college and came home, so a lodger it must be. I had discussed it with him and told him that I was making a start by getting a home that would be 'ours' when he left college, somewhere to start our life together, somewhere to live when we got married. He seemed happy to begin with. Then he began, as usual, to spread his blackness, and deflate my elation. He found fault in every single thing about it: where it was, how it looked, how big it was, the list went on. When it came to moving in and decorating, he was no-where to be seen, didn't want to help with what was going to be his house too, just didn't care. Didn't want to know. Then once I had struggled with moving and decorating and sorting things out, he suddenly appeared, was less busy with some time to spend there. He sat in the armchair in the lounge with his feet on the table, like he was a king, triumphant, the master of all he surveyed. His serfs had done all of the work. It was amazing how much he seemed to enjoy the house once I had done everything by myself. I was angry and fed up. Fed up with his drinking, fed up with his anger, and fed up with constantly being undermined. He began to sense I was not happy, and kept asking and asking if I was okay, but I pretended I was fine. It was the pressures of school, I would say. In reality I was scared of the way he would react, or what he might do if I told him I wasn't happy or if I told him that maybe we would be better apart. He began to drop things into conversation, like he would never let me go, he'd always come after me, and that he'd kill himself if we ever split up. And I became more and more anxious. The more I tried to distance myself the more frightening and irrational he became. I vividly remember one Sunday afternoon, that we sat together on the sofa reading the Sunday papers. He was reading a profile of a man who had gone into an infant school classroom and had stabbed and killed many of the children there, then had stabbed and killed the teacher. He looked up from the crumpled article, dark and blazing underneath a veil of calmness, and with intense piercing eyes stared through me.

"I can relate to this man," he said in seriousness. My face drained and paled with shock.

"He must be joking," I thought. He was not.

"These things in his childhood I can relate to," he continued. "I know how he feels." He looked deep into my eyes, waiting for a reaction,

"Don't worry," he smiled. "I would never hurt any children..."

I understood perfectly what he meant, maybe not the children, just the teacher, just me. He carried on reading the paper and I sat there in terrified, silent solitude, pretending everything was okay.

Our relationship carried on being rough for months, and I was still too terrified to finish it for a sack-full of reasons. The Summer Ball was upon us once more at his college, the one I had previously been to for four years. I was excited, yet nervous. We were going to try and make it romantic, make it special, really make an effort to put things right. I was looking forward to it with anxious anticipation as I hurriedly drove straight from school, to the college, with my ball gown laid carefully on the back seat of the car. I had hung it in the corner of the classroom all day so as not to let it get too creased, and the children thought it was wonderful. They all wanted to see me in it. They all thought I was going to be a beautiful fairy princess. They kept on at me all day to put it on, so Mrs Pike the reception class teacher sat both of our classes on the carpet and said she was going to do something magical and turn me into a princess. She got all of the children to close their eyes tight and make a wish to make the magic work, and as they did I slipped out of the classroom and put on my dress. When the children opened their eyes there I was, Miss Williams, the fairy princess. They all squealed with delight and excitement. They still believed in fairytales and magic, and I wished with all my heart that I still did as I stood there in my red satin meringue, with messy hair, spots and muddy work makeup. They didn't see the flaws, they only saw the beauty; children always did. We have a lot to learn from them.

Hoping I would still feel like a princess that night, I raced up the iron staircase in the halls of residence, bags and dress in hand, to Phil's room. I pressed the buzzer and, as the door swung open, Phil's brother's girlfriend, who was in a black satin gown, greeted me. I was amazed; I had no idea that she or Mike had been invited. I gulped back my shock, pretending I knew all about them coming, and asked where the boys were.

"Phil asked me to wait here for you, they've gone to the pub and will pick us up on the way back." My heart sank as my stomach rose into my mouth. He was drinking already, he had promised he wouldn't, and I could see the evening panning out bleakly before me.

When they eventually came back we made our way across the tree-lined campus towards the main college building. It was an old grey stone building which stood proudly overlooking rolling green hills and woodlands and down into the valley beyond. I had often sat, and looked, and thought, that maybe the view was a beautiful painted stage set that someone had propped up at the edge of the gardens and forgotten to put away. It seemed so beautifully serene and magnificent it was hard to believe it was real. The college was over two hundred years old and looked imposing and strong, and had a huge stone staircase lined with unusually fragrant pink roses sweeping up to the entrance. Above the entrance to the college stood the clock tower with its large blue face and glittering golden numerals, and right at the top of the tower, on a bright white flag pole, hung the welsh dragon. It flew high and flapped proudly against the sky's purples and reds and blues which had all melted and mixed together as the last fingers of sunlight glowed and caressed the horizon, and the excited chatter of students past and present filled the warm summer sky. I had had such a special time here, and I dreamed of the good times, the fun times, the friendships, and the happy, happy memories as we swept along. And I was filled with tremendous joy at being back on such a romantic occasion.

We entered the huge red and white candy striped marquee to a chorus of 'Rachael!!!' being screamed across from the bar. Everyone ran over and Jack picked me up then whizzed and spun me around cheerfully, my poppy skirt puffing and billowing its layers of petals up into the air. All of the gang were there, and I hadn't seen many of them since we had gone our separate ways the previous year. I grabbed Phil by the hand and on our behalf introduced all of them to Mike and Maggie. It was so lovely to see them all again. I turned to give Phil an excited kiss and stopped myself in shock. His lips were tight, his face was tight and his eyes looked as if they were going to explode out of his head with burning anger. I couldn't understand what was wrong, except that he was already beginning to turn into a beery monster. Surely he wasn't angry at me for introducing my friends to Mike and Maggie. Even he couldn't be jealous about that. Then it hit me. He had invited Mike and Maggie over to show just how 'popular' he was and what a 'cool' time he was having. But the reality was different. He hadn't made any real friends there since he had begun a year ago. That wasn't my fault though, was it? What was I supposed to do, hide in the corner, not speak to anyone, and pretend that he was God and the centre of the universe and nobody else existed? No, this couldn't be happening, it would be far too childish. Then I thought that maybe I was imagining it all, he'd be calmer in a minute, and maybe it was all in my head, which by now was whirling around madly. I needed a break to gather my thoughts, so I excused myself politely and headed to the ladies room. On the way back I bumped into Will and Keith, the two college security guards who were in their sixties. I was very fond of them both and had spent a lot of time with them when I worked on the college switchboard in the evenings. We had had a really fun time on the reception desk together, and it was lovely to see them again. We all caught up on the news, views and gossip, and smiling I went back to Phil, his brother and Maggie. Phil's mood had darkened still, his face frowned and his eyes glowered menacingly.

"Where have you been?" he hissed in my ear so as no-one could see or hear, and held my wrist tightly.

"I've been to the ladies, then I bumped into Will and Keith and had a chat, it was really good to see them," I smiled, trying to crack the stormy atmosphere.

"Why didn't you take me with you?" his grip became tighter.

"You couldn't come into the ladies with me, and then I bumped into them. I could hardly come back and drag you away from the others and leave Mike and Maggie on their own could I?" I was now wincing from the pressure of his grip on my wrist.

"You just don't get it do you?" He spat viciously into my face. I could feel his venom boiling up inside him, and he was right, I didn't get it. He let go of my wrist, picked up his beer and turned his back on me. My jaw dropped and I blinked back the tears that were beginning to saltily sting my eyes. So much for our romantic evening! I tried to pretend that nothing was wrong, and joined in with the laughter and the gaiety of the evening. I tried to chat happily to Phil, but each time I tried he blanked me completely and continued to acquaint himself with his amber liquid friend. At last dinner was to be served, so we all made our way into the college dining room which had been magnificently transformed into a luxurious restaurant. There were crisp white tablecloths, flickering white candles on golden holders that twinkled with the fluttering flickers, and bowls of pink carnations and gypsophila on every table, and everything looked magical. There were even proper white plates and heavy, hired cutlery. I was mesmerised. The meal was beautiful, and obviously not cooked in the college canteen, and we all chatted and laughed. Phil was including me again now that we were with company, and I felt everything was going to be just fine. When the meal was finished Phil smilingly left the table, and I followed behind him. He had been drinking all through the meal but seemed fine, so I felt a little easier. When we got outside into the corridor his smile fell and smashed onto the floor and he pulled away from me angrily. I quickened my pace as best I could and tip tapping, tottered after him down the corridor.

"Phil I'm sorry," I pleaded as I caught him up. "I'm really, really sorry for whatever it is I've done to upset you so much. Come on, let's have a lovely night together, I don't want you to be angry."

He flew around and grabbed both of my arms so tightly that they began to throb as his fingers sunk deeply into my flesh.

He was boiling and bubbling behind his eyes.

"You really don't know what you've done wrong do you?" he sneered.

"No I don't. Please tell me, I don't understand. Whatever it is, I'm really, really sorry. Come on let's have a nice night," I pleadingly smiled, but it came out wonky as the confusion and fear twisted and screwed it up.

"You just don't fucking understand what you've done wrong. If you can't work it out," he slurred. "I'm not going to tell you." And he pushed me aside and lurched away. I still didn't understand, and I was so confused and upset and frightened. So I decided, right there and then, that there was no way I was going to spend the night with the monster when he was in this state. So I went to my security guard friends and explained what was happening. They were all for having a word with him and sorting it out, but I said that all I wanted them to do was to unlock his room with the master key, so that I could get my things out and put them in my car. Keith walked me over to Phil's room, steadying my arm as we went, and stood and watched as I grabbed my bags, making sure I was okay. He carried them to my car, like a real gentleman, and heaved them into the back for me. I thanked him tearfully for his help and for getting me out of a really horrid predicament, and softly kissed his cheek. He had always been so kind to me. I felt relieved that whatever happened that evening, at least I would be able to go home.

I went back into the dark hall and swam through a heaving sea of partying people, who were all bobbing up and down in time to the band, their faces appearing and disappearing as the lights caught them luminously in mid-boogie. And the faces were all laughing and smiling as they turned off and on like hundreds of lighthouse warnings, warning me of my impending doom. And everyone except me seemed to be having a fantastic time. The girls were sleek and shiny, or layered in flounces, with a myriad of colours and sparkles, and the boys were all black and white, amazingly smart and looked like bobby-dazzlers. It never ceased to amaze me how the boys, who were such smelly, scruffy students, could scrub up to be so smart and dashing and handsome. The power of the tuxedo! I spotted Phil and the others and went over. I tried again to talk to Phil but he blanked me each time I tried. He danced around and around me like I wasn't even there, with his own menacing war dance. The room throbbed, the beat of the drum grew strong and loud, and I stood there in the cooking pot. I knew he could get funny, but I would never have expected this, I was so upset I didn't know what to do. And still he danced around and around me, and still I wasn't there. Now I knew how a handbag felt. I wasn't going to put up with this, I wasn't going to stand there and be continually humiliated by his ignorance. So I kept going off and chatting to my friends, then coming back to see if he'd calmed down, which he hadn't, and on and on it went. My friends, especially the boys, were really angry with him and wanted to go and sort him out. They couldn't believe what was going on. But I wouldn't let them get involved as I knew how nasty he could be, and I certainly didn't want them getting into trouble because of me.

"How dare he treat you like this, it's disgraceful," Howard fumed. "You should never treat a lady like this. Especially a lady who's my friend." He was really angry. They all were. I carried on trying to get Phil to even acknowledge my existence, let alone speak to me, but it was no good. He just danced around and around in circles, swaying and stumbling and barging into me, with sweat pouring down his face and with his wobbling pint in his hand. Judging by the state of his once white shirt, he had spilt as much on him as he had drunk. I didn't need this, and I didn't deserve this. It was coming to the end of the night and I was going home. I went up to Mike and Maggie, and apologised and said I hoped that what had happened hadn't spoilt the evening too much for them, and that I wasn't sure what was going on or what I had done wrong. And I was really surprised by Mike's reaction. The once loyal brother said he couldn't believe the way that Phil had treated me all evening.

"I know he's my brother, and I thought I knew him even though he's spent a lot of time at sea, but I don't know him at all. I'm really ashamed of him. I'm really sorry that you've had such a crap time, I've tried talking some sense into him but I really don't know what the hell's wrong with him. I've never seen him like this before and I really wouldn't blame you if you finished with him, but I really, really hope you don't. Please Rach, don't finish it." His eyes pleaded with me.

"Look Mike, I'm not putting up with this any more. I don't know what I'm going to do, but I'm not staying with him tonight. Thanks for your support anyway." I smiled at them both and worked my way through the crowd and headed along the lonely dark corridor, leaving the lights and the music and the fun-filled party behind me. I could hear footsteps following me, thundery, stumbling footsteps, and an angry voice shouting and shouting. I ignored it but it carried on shouting and shouting. I turned around and there he was, beer stained and lurching from side to side like he was still rolling about on his ship.

"We need to talk," he slurred.

"Fine. Lets go somewhere quieter." He stumbled determinedly behind me as I led him to the deserted cafeteria, where a few people hung around in clumps, looking worn out and weary as they chatted and drank, away from the noise and the crowds and the flashing lights.

"Right talk," I said. I was boiling mad underneath my calm exterior, and I was trembling. Trembling with rage and fear, anger and disbelief. This was it, his chance, his last chance, his one and only chance. He had a lot of apologising to do before I would or could ever forgive him. He pointed his finger into my chest and stabbed and poked and jab, jab, jabbed.

" It's your fault I'm like this, you're such a bitch, you don't care, you just do what you want....." he spat and dribbled as he shouted into my face. "You don't realise what you've done, you make me angry, your friends...you're such a bitch, you don't get it..." He was angry and rambling and making no sense. I tried so hard to understand him, but I just couldn't make out what he was trying to say through the slurring spitting venom. And I could see him beginning to inflate like a poisonous balloon, and one look, one word, one move would make him explode in my face. It was time to go. I thought he might have wanted to talk and apologise for making me look so stupid all night and behaving so cruelly and irrationally. But no, he just wanted to shout and swear and try to scare me; but this time, it was not going to work. I got up off the chair, took a deep breath, and drew myself up tall and proud and strong, summoning up every ounce of strength and courage that

I had. Inside I was trembling like a jelly in an earthquake.

"I am not staying here to have you speak to me like this. You're being nasty, and you're not making any sense, so I'm going. Ring me in the morning when you're sober." I turned and slowly walked away.

He began shouting at me. "Don't you walk away from me...don't you dare walk away from me!" I began to panic. I could hear anger in his voice and could hear him stumbling after me. My footsteps quickened and my heart began to race. I could feel the balloon getting larger and larger, as I got quicker and quicker.

"Ring me when you're sober, ring me when you're sober," I repeated again and again, trying to keep myself calm, and trying to make him realise that this was the end of the conversation, but he would not give up. As I raced away I was swept along by the sea of people who had finished dancing and were washing out of the hall and floating along the corridor. As I doggy paddled along I could hear the thunderous bang of the balloon exploding into a thousand pieces, and I could see it shooting lightening above and over the heads of the crowd. And the hot air rushed screaming out, getting louder and louder and louder.

"You walk away from me now you fucking bitch, you walk away from me now and that's it, it's fucking over...You fucking walk away from me now and it's fucking over....." He was a hysterical screaming tidal wave crashing over the heads of the sea of bobbing people, trying desperately to drown me with his bullying anger.

But I could feel my strength rising and rising, and swelling and swelling, and all of the good memories and the good friends that I had had there filled me with courage and strength and love. If I couldn't do it here, I would never ever be able to do it. So I took a deep breath and with my head held high I walked away. I walked away through the throngs of happy tiddly people all chatting and laughing, through the old and friendly buildings I knew so well and out into the fresh air, as fast as I could. I left him to drown.

I got into my tiny mini, changed my heels for my Dr Marten boots, and drove away with my chin resting on the top of my puffed up red ball gown. Away, away, away and home. I looked as if I was sitting in the middle of an inflated parachute as I drove along, but I just didn't care. I just wanted to get away. I think he thought I had to stay, had to put up with him, and had to put up with his vile abuse. But he hadn't realised that I had stopped drinking five hours before and that all of my things were now in my car, so I could no longer be held to ransom. I was glad I had sixth sense. So I drove and drove, deep into the darkness, away from him, away from his anger, away from his drinking, away, away, away.

He thought I would ring him. I always did. Always did to keep the peace and to smooth things over, even when I had done nothing wrong. And that was most of the time. Always tried to keep things calm, it was easier that way. This time I vowed I wouldn't go crawling to him. I never saw him again. Never found out what was wrong and never found out what had happened. But at last I was free. It had been such a horrendous night but at least I knew I had done nothing wrong, it was not my fault, and many others had seen a part of him that they never knew was there, the part that I had known about for a long, long time.

Although we were apart it took a long time for him to be exorcised. I was terrified he would come and get me while in one of his irrational and angry drunken rages. I remembered all of the threats; they raced around inside my head and left me sleeping restlessly for months. I slept each night with a knife under my pillow, just in case. Each creak, each rustle, each click I heard, I would hold my breath and listen. Listen to make sure it wasn't him, he wasn't there, he hadn't come to get me. Night after night I waited, but thankfully he never came. And sometimes I would sit and gaze out of my classroom window at the grass and the trees and the sky, and plan what I was going to do if he did come to get me at school. I planned scenarios and escape routes and what I would do to defeat him if he came into my classroom. I remembered all of the things that he had said, all of his threats, and all of the innuendoes. But as time went by they began to fade like a shop window display in the sun, and I began to live my life again.

I went out with two men after Phil, and both of them came with their problems. One came with a cannabis and cocaine habit, and the other came with an alcohol problem and a touch of six month amnesia, where he had forgotten to tell me that he had a wife and an eleven year old daughter in another town. I always seemed to pick the wrong men, and I always put up with what ever they had to throw at me. It all seemed so ridiculous and humiliating when I heard myself telling Sylvia about the dreadful relationships that I had managed to become entangled in. If I had heard anyone else telling her about such a dreadful time, I would have told them in no uncertain terms that they were foolish and should finish the disastrous and destructive relationship immediately. I felt really, really stupid, and I was angry with myself. What on earth was wrong with me? I thought hard about why I kept choosing such dreadful men, and why I kept accepting the unacceptable.

Slowly it began to dawn on me. I kept choosing the wrong men because I didn't think that I deserved someone who was decent and loving and kind. I thought that someone like that would never want me, why should they want someone as horrid as me when there were so many beautiful and wonderful women out there. That was the trouble, I felt worthless, dirty and ugly, so I thought that only men with some kind of problem of their own would want me. And once I got into a relationship which had major problems, I would accept them because I believed that no-one else would want me or like me, so I had better stick with the dreadful relationship that I had, rather than risk being unwanted and unloved for ever. I felt that if I met a man who needed me in some way, I would be able to help him, and he wouldn't be able to do without me. I felt that if he couldn't do without me, then he would never leave me, he would need me, no matter how ugly or disgusting I was. I also felt that if I was with someone who had a problem, then no-one else would want to be with them, as no normal person would put up with the baggage that they brought, and they would realise this and stay with me.

It was ridiculous the way that I saw things, and I was amazed when I looked inside my head at how my crazy mind was with regard to relationships. It was crazy and contradictory. Because although I wanted to be with someone and for them to never leave me, I also think deep, deep inside, I felt that if I chose someone who was 'wrong', then I would never be totally close to them, and if I was never totally close to them, then I could never be hurt in the way that I was hurt by Dean. He tore my heart in two. It was really odd, it seemed that I had convinced myself that it was normal to have a relationship that made me feel bad, and that it was totally inconceivable that somewhere out there, there might actually be a nice man, with no problems, who loved me and would never hurt me. I really didn't think that that could ever be possible. And the reason that I thought that it would never be possible, was because I felt so awful about myself. I was ugly and worthless and unlovable, so I felt I had to accept any old crap that came my way. I also felt that I had to please everyone and make everyone like me, so the more horrible and hurtful a partner became towards me; the more I tried to do the right thing and make them like me, it was madness, utter madness. At least I was beginning to see that now. The blackness had destroyed every droplet of confidence and self-worth and self-belief that I had ever had, and so I had to begin to truly love myself before I would ever find someone who truly loved me. I realised that this sounded corny, but Sylvia agreed with everything that I said. She placed her warm, smooth hand upon mine and told me she was going to give me some homework. She told me that I had to look into the mirror every day, and deep into my own eyes and tell myself 'I love you,' at least ten times a day. "How embarrassing! How ridiculous!" I thought.

But when I got home I began to do my homework task as soon as I walked through the door. It was really,

really difficult, and I felt incredibly foolish, and terribly fraudulent. I didn't love myself. I wasn't worth anybody's love, let alone my own. But I battled with myself, and tried and tried to do it. I would sit cross legged on my bedroom floor and struggle to lift my eyes up from the pale blue carpet and look at the stranger that peeked sheepishly back at me from the wardrobe mirror.

"I love you," I would mutter, staring at the red spot shining at me from my chin, or the dull, drab hair roots that were now betraying me as the fraud that I was. Not able to look into my own eyes. Not able to convince myself that I did love me, and that I deserved to be loved. But every day I battled until one day I met the stare of the stranger in the mirror, looked deep, deep into her eyes and told her "I love you," and meant it. And the stranger smiled back at me with a warm glow on her cheeks and a faint twinkle in her eyes, and the moment passed and the blackness flooded back. But each time I made the stranger glow it lasted longer and longer, and I think in the end she began to believe me, and she smiled back as she passed me a pebble, "I love you too."

CHAPTER FOURTEEN

I sat on the cold tiles of the kitchen floor surrounded by boxes of this and that. The two cats paced around and around, sniffing and rubbing the boxes and letting out meows of angst as they flicked their tails in agitation. I couldn't let them out of the kitchen as the removal men were removing the boxes and bags and things from the house, and were stacking them with military precision into the enormous white removal van. They came to get the last few boxes from the kitchen, and I hung on to the somersaulting cats. Then leaving the cats in the kitchen, and shutting the door carefully behind me, I went and watched the last pieces being fitted into the huge and complicated puzzle. It didn't bother me, seeing all of the furniture and the boxes containing all of our lives piled up, pushed in, and slotted together. I was so used to having my life in a box it seemed quite normal, but this time it wasn't sadness and misfortune that had us packing our things away, we were just moving on, moving up, moving to a new and better place. They slid the heavy steel doors shut, locked them secure, and drove down the road, around the corner and away to the new beginning. It didn't even bother me seeing all of our things disappearing into the distance, as I had already lost everything, and had come to realise that the only thing you really have in your life is yourself. And the only things that matter in your life are your real friends, your family, love, happiness and most importantly your health. I had the first two, and I was working hard to achieve three, four and five. I went back into the empty shell of what used to be the family home and wandered around each echoey room saying good-bye and remembering the fun, the sadness, the laughter, the tears, the rows and the reconciliations, which all rolled themselves into a bundle and called themselves family life. We had lived here for a long time, and as a little tear leaked out I said my good-byes and smiled. It was time to move on, it was time to start afresh, it was time to say good-bye to the old, and time to begin building the foundations of a new life.

My mum had thought that moving would be far too traumatic for me in my present condition, so she had given me one, and only one, important job to do. I had to look after and bring the cats. I pushed open the kitchen door gingerly, putting my foot in the crack to deter any fluffy, angry critters from making a bid for freedom and slid myself through the door. They were still storming around the now empty kitchen and every so often frantically scratching at the locked cat-flap hoping it might just give way and let them propel themselves into freedom. I picked up Marmite the pampered black fluffy one, with tiny feet and a tiny face and a huge Basil Brush fluffy tail, and tried to put her into her carrying basket. Her legs stuck out in all directions, rigid and waving in prison-evading swimming manoeuvres. As I folded each leg in, in turn, the others would all pop out and wave around as she wriggled and squiggled and I rolled around on the floor trying with all my might to push the star-shaped cat into the square-shaped hole. Eventually, after a battle of wits and great feats of strength, I managed to squish the stroppy, scratchy, biting, bugger into the basket and tether the door shut. And to my amazement, I only sustained two open running wounds and one excellent dental impression that was good enough for a forensic dentist to use in case she ever needed identifying. And if she carried on like that again she might just need identifying. The deceptively kind-natured sweetie looked terrified, and her huge, winkingly-wide green eyes stared out from behind the bars as she huddled at the back of the basket in frozen terror. I turned triumphant and bleeding to face Poppy, the feisty, spitty, angry tortoiseshell who was now eying me up scarily from the corner of the room and sneering as she weighed up exactly how much blood she was going to spill, and licked her lips. I slowly rolled down the sleeves of my thick black jumper, until my arms and my hands and my fingers were covered with pathetic, penetrable protection. Who was I kidding! I bent down slowly towards Poppy who had backed herself into the corner and had turned herself into a hissing, spitting, coiled viper, shuddering and shaking and ready to strike. I lowered my hands slowly towards her, keeping my face well back from the slashy, bitey bits and lifted her up. She looked at me with an expression of passive surrender, then shrugged her shoulders and turned into a limp and lollopy lettuce. "Okay, it's a fair cop," she purred as I plopped her passively into the basket. I was flabbergasted; I didn't need an ambulance! I was amazed at how the cat's characters changed when they were frightened, and that they didn't react in the ways in which I thought they both would, to what they saw as a frightening situation. When I thought about it humans were the same, you never know how you will react to a frightening situation until you're in one, so you couldn't ever really judge other people's reactions to bad situations. Fight, flight, freeze, or fidget about, the choice is yours. It was the same for animals and humans alike. I carried the two jumpy carriers to my car and put them on the back seats. I went back up the front path and stood and looked up at the house. It seemed so familiar, so comforting, so safe, with its red bricks, and its pinky-yellow flowered honeysuckle growing over the top of the sturdy porch, which kept life's rain from falling on your head. And as I looked it seemed as though it was bulging at the seams with memories, like an over-full, musty, brown photo album, and it seemed as if it was about to burst and flutter the photos all over the garden. We had, at last, outgrown it, and it was time to move on and create some new memories somewhere else, somewhere where there was more space to breathe, and more space to grow. The house shuddered and heaved an empty sigh as I slammed the heavy, dark, wooden front door on the past, walked down the path and drove away to a new beginning.

I arrived at the new house too soon to bring the cats in as the men were still heaving and hauling the boxes and bags and furniture off the back of the van and dispersing it according to the cleverly organised labels my mother had placed on everything. The driveway was blocked and swarming with men and vans and cars and my father and his harassed and tired-out face, so I drove along the road and parked in the car park of the tyre and exhaust garage. The cats by now were squawking and singing with voices like tight violin strings, so I decided to sing as well to calm them down. The only songs that came to me were songs from the bits of my happy childhood, so the cats enjoyed a variety of Abba medleys. And soon their singing stopped as they stared, mew-less and mutely mesmerised, as they both tried to absorb the tunelessness of the songs and the made up nonsensical words I had invented to fill the gaps in the lyrics, which I couldn't remember. We sat there for ages, and all the time I carried on singing Abba songs, and the cats seemed calm and listened. I didn't sing Waterloo though as I thought that might be tempting bottom tinkling fate. As the men in the tyre garage wandered past the open doors, in greasy once-blue overalls, they chuckled at the sight of the mad girl in the car singing to herself. But I had to sing, as I was singing to calm all three of us, Marmite, Poppy and me. We all trembled in the car at the prospect of the strange new house, and the start of a strange new life, so we all sang, and we all felt better.

When I saw the last of the large white removal vans pull out from the red brick driveway and head off in the direction of the nearest bacon butty van, I drove myself and the cats through the fir tree fence and parked outside our new house. It was large, brand spanking new, made from Cotswold stone, and had a new sturdy porch to protect you from life's rain. To the right of the house was a tiny stream and a brambly hedge, behind which were the massively spacious grounds of The Manor House. Large trees lined the brambly hedge and stooped over the house, protecting it from the outside world. To the left of the house was a reflection of our house, exactly the same but back to front, and beyond that were other large houses all tucked behind the fir tree fence, then the road built up a little as it swept into the heart of the village. I lifted the two bouncing boxes from the back of the car and took them around to the utility room, where mum had already laid out their wicker baskets with garishly colourful crochet blankets, their food and water bowls, litter trays and a selection of teddy bears. I'm not sure for whose benefit the teddies were, probably to alleviate my mother's guilt at the upheaval for the cats, but they lined up along the worktop like a smiley welcoming committee. I shut the doors to the utility room and opened the doors to the cat carriers, then sat on the floor and waited for the wide-eyed creatures to investigate. Poppy hurtled out and around and around in circles, bouncing like a Tigger and trying to hurl herself at the window on the top half of the back door, thinking it was a viable escape route. Marmite quaked in the darkness at the back of the basket and was eventually coaxed out by tender words and lullabies, sniffed around trembling and leaving little footprints of nervous sweat on the worktops, before curling up in denial in her familiar basket with her purple teddy. Poppy, after extensive exploration of the small utility room and all of its corners, curled up in a purring unrecognisable bundle on my lap and went to sleep. She felt safe with me, and as I took the rare opportunity to gently stroke the top of her ginger flecked head, I felt relieved. We were all here, we were all safe, we would all be okay.

As the evening began to draw in the house had already become settled and unpacked, due my mothers amazing organisation and determination, so I went out into the cool air of the back garden. I walked across the soft lawn and stood at the bottom of the garden, resting my elbows on the top of the ranch fence that separated me from the meadow, the fields, and the rolling sheep-dappled hills beyond. The air was crisp and clean and the night's first stars began to twinkle above me. Two tiny, whizzy, black bats darted past each other and all around, far faster than I could watch them. They zoomed and zig-zagged and flitted with amazing aeronautical prowess, the like of which I had never seen. I thought to myself that they looked liked mini spacecrafts and I was sure that the air force would do anything to be able to manoeuvre their aeroplanes like that. Nothing ever makes me marvel quite as much as the fantastical things found in nature. I stood and watched them play until the darkness had crept all over the sky and dipped down behind the hills. I was numb and scared and confused with everything in my life, but I smiled as the pure fresh air softly tingled in my nose and began to cleanse me on the inside. I shivered a little as I made my way back inside and up the stairs to my new bedroom. I had decided I wanted everything in it to be cream, to be clean, to be fresh. I thought that if I began to surround myself with beautiful things, and fresh things, then it would maybe begin to cleanse and refresh me on the inside. I began to make my bed up. I had bought myself all brand new, cream embroidered bed linen, pillow cases and sheets, and I had kept them all wrapped up and unused until we moved to the new house. I had even bought myself a new pair of pyjamas with pretty pink rose buds on, and I had decided that I was going to brainwash myself into thinking that I was new and clean and pretty too. It had been an extremely tiring and stressful day, but instead of crawling straight into bed like I would have done before, I sunk myself down into a deep, bubbly, lily-scented bath. I lay there for ages letting the dirt seep out and the beautiful sweet scent seep in, and I traced the ceiling of the unfamiliar bathroom with my eyes. I dreamed and drifted as the warmth caressed me and soothed the edges of the sadness away.

I slipped between the crisp new sheets, wearing the crisp new pyjamas, smelling of lovely lilies, and smiled to myself. I was still desperately ill, but at least I had a fresh new start, a chance to start my life again.

My bedroom became my sanctuary, all fresh and cream and new and beautiful. And I always made sure that I had fresh and fragrant flowers in there, upon the windowsill in clear view, so that I could always see them. If I made it calm and beautiful, then maybe it would make me calm and beautiful. But every night, without exception, the night time demons would come rampaging back and I would wake up screaming and drowning in sweat, as my mother burst through the doors to rescue me. And she would cradle me in her arms and stroke my brow and try to soothe the terror away, as she did when I was a child, and she would sing my favourite lullaby, softly and sweetly. And every night I went to bed so utterly exhausted that I was sure I was never going to wake up again. I was convinced I was going to die, right there and then in my own beautiful bed. And I would cry and quake with fear as my mother tried desperately to comfort me, each and every night. I may have been able to try and banish the dirt and the blackness from my room during the day, but as soon as I shut my eyelids at night and drifted quietly into sleep, every monster, every demon, every devil would all scream out from the darkness and torture and maim, then bite, slash and tear me, until I woke up screaming myself hoarse and tearfully terrified. It was so horrific that sometimes I just didn't want to close my eyes, just didn't want to sleep, as I couldn't face the horror of the demonic nightmares. So my mum would often sit with me in the gentle glow of the nightlight, and wait for me to fall into a peaceful sleep before she would creep out of my room, and back into her own. I guess my brain was trying to resolve my pain and mend itself, and this disturbing and terrifying debris was the result. But I hoped and prayed that it wouldn't go on forever.

CHAPTER FIFTEEN

I smiled as I told Sylvia all about our new house and how lovely it was, and how quiet and peaceful it was, and how the air was fresh and pure and cleansing. And how every afternoon when I felt the same old overwhelming urge to sleep, I would go down to the bottom of the garden and lie on my back on a warm woollen blanket. And I would stare up at the dappled light that was sprinkling like icing sugar through the leaves of the trees and would listen as the leaves softly swished in the breeze, like the sea lapping and gently rippling on the shore. And I would take in long, deep breaths of the warm fresh air that tasted of minty honeysuckle it was so fresh and sweet, and quietly I would slip into peaceful, smiley sleep. The demons mostly seemed to visit at night, so I would sleep softly until a bird's boisterous, jolly song, or an inquisitive cat rubbing her furry cheek along my face would wake me up. Sylvia smiled as she steered my problem displacing conversation in the direction of today's counselling session. A furrow ploughed its way across my brow, these sessions were traumatic and difficult, but I knew they were beginning to help, and I knew I had to unload my self before I could ever wipe my slate clean and begin my life again.

I had begun to suffer from spots in my teenage years, as most teenagers do. But mine always seemed worse to me than everyone else's, and I was quite embarrassed by them. I tried to take no notice of them, but they always made me feel slightly dirty and unattractive. I put up with them for a couple of years as I thought they were part of teenage life, but as they got more and more on top of me I went to the doctor; the first of many trips to the doctor. He looked at them, didn't say an awful lot, and gave me some cream. I was pleased and hoped it would work. This farcical loop went on for years, managing, going to the doctors, being given some different cream or lotion or potion, and going home full of hope. Full of hope that maybe, just maybe, this time it would actually work. Then after months of persevering and it not working I would give up. I was quite self-conscious and I was already feeling bad enough about myself, so the spots were the icing on the cake. I thought I would grow out of them, as most kids do, but as my friends' complexions began to clear leaving them with peachy, beautiful skin, mine stayed the same. I hated it. And it just went on and on and on. I went to the college doctor when I went away to live, to see if he had a solution, but he bundled me away with another solution 'dab it on, you'll be fine,' he said. I was not fine. I was in my twenties now, and still they shone there for all to see. I was so self-conscious and they made me feel so ugly, that I was sure people thought I must spend all of my time eating chips and chocolate and not washing. I was convinced that's what people thought. And it chipped away, bit by bit, the little confidence that I did have with men. Who would want an ugly spotty girlfriend when they could have a peach? I battled with it at college with my lotions and my cunning disguising make-up, and I bubbled out exuberance hoping no-one would notice that underneath the froth I still had the skin of a fifteen year old. When I left college I began teaching, and my spots began to get worse. I would spend each day feeling tense and embarrassed as I knew everyone could see the blemishes bulging from underneath my concealing spot stick. I would start to worry and become upset as I could feel a new one begin to pulsate and throb and feel it engulf the whole of my face, or so it felt. At every opportunity I would race to the toilets with spot stick in hand, to check on my face's progress and to try and dab, dab, dab a disguise on any spots that had begun to burst through. It got so bad that on a Friday night I would heave a sigh of relief, I was so glad I didn't have to see anyone until Monday, and that no-one could see my face until then. I would sit in the bathroom on a Friday night after I had had a shower and washed away the disguise, and stare despairingly into the mirror. The redness would shine back at me and my face would be throbbing, so that even if I couldn't see the spots I could feel them all of the time. All of the time. I would rest my head in my hands and cry as I eyed up the mess that was my face, and it became so distressing for me that I would often phone up friends to excuse myself from the weekend festivities as I would be feeling too upset and far too self conscious to join in. I just wanted to hide until they all went away. But they never went away.

One Friday night I phoned for a delivery pizza, I always found it mildly amusing, a pepperoni pizza ordering a pepperoni pizza, and I sat and waited for it with a glass of wine in hand. I flicked through one of those glossy, 'you can and you must have it all or you're a failure', women's magazines, and from it fell a little white foil packet, which plopped onto my lap. I eyed it suspiciously, then read the label carefully, as usually the samples given away with most magazines were pointless and useless and you wouldn't buy the product in a million years. That was probably where the free samples came from, the mountains of leftover bottles of jollop, which they couldn't shift. And the contents of these bottles were funnelled into tiny little foil packages and given away free in the vain hope that someone would like, and maybe even buy, the gungy pungent potion. The little white packet that had found its way onto my lap was a new, super-dooper foundation called 'Perfect', and allegedly it would disguise all of your blemishes and pimples, and warts and spots, and make you look and feel perfect and beautiful again. I laughed, what a load of cobblers. 'Oh well,' I thought. 'I'm bored waiting for the pizza so I might as well give it a go for a laugh.' I went upstairs to the bathroom, pulled on the florescent light over the bathroom mirror and eyed the mess that was my face. 'I think I need Merlin, not make-up,' I thought as I inspected the throbbing red mass. I tore off the top of the pouch with my teeth and squeezed the miracle makeup onto my finger. It was the colour of someone who had overdosed on poor quality fake tan, but I began to smear it on in some vain and desperate hope that it might just work and cover the monstrosity that was me. As I began to smear it over the contours of my face I couldn't believe my eyes, the spots that I had seemed to begin to disappear and leave me with an even, if somewhat tangerine coloured skin. When I had finished I stood back and looked at my now even complexion. It might still be lumpy and bumpy, but at least it was all the same colour. I was always convinced that if you wore foundation it would block your pores and make spots worse, but after all these years of being embarrassed and ashamed I really didn't care any more. The next day I rushed out to the chemist and bought a bottle of this wonder potion, in the right colour this time, and put it straight on. It made me feel a little better, a little less self-conscious, a little more attractive. But still the spots stayed. I wore the makeup every day, and when I had a partner, every night. I would go into the bathroom to take my makeup off ready for bed, take off all of the day makeup, have a wash, then put only the foundation back on so that it looked as though I had taken everything off, and my ugly secret remained just that, a secret. I was so embarrassed by my skin that I was sure it would send men running and screaming if they ever caught me without my make up on. The battle still continued.

As I was getting much healthier, by eating healthily and going to the gym at least four times a week, I thought I needed to try to find a natural remedy, a healthy alternative to the chemicals I kept being given by the doctor. So I made an appointment to see a Chinese herbalist. I found it amazing when I got there that the clinic was situated in one of the most run down, congested and busy streets in the city. As I walked towards it I was jostled and hustled by grey people all pushing and shoving, wearing angry faces and cheap nylon clothes, and it seemed that all of them had fags permanently dangling from the corners of their mouths. And they were all inhaling the billowing clouds of grey fumes being spat out of the backs of the queues of multicoloured metallic beasts. I wondered how somewhere that was supposed to be one of the healthiest healing places around could exist in such a dirty stinking hole, and then I realised why. The people here needed more help than most to keep themselves healthy as they were being contaminated every day from the fumes, and poisoned by each other and by themselves. I stood outside the clinic and read the various ailments that they claimed to cure, all printed naively and quite crudely on the glass of the window in large red letters. It seemed that they could cure all kinds of aches and pains and lumps and bumps and eczema and headaches and all sorts of things including helping to give up smoking; which the locals had obviously not taken up. I hoped they would be able to help me too. I swished open the glass door and entered the clinic, and it was like entering a different and very exotic world. An unusual smell hit my nose, and it was unlike anything else I had ever smelt. It was a musty, herby, spicy smell, unusually unrecognisable and strong. There was no-one in the shop, so I stood patiently and waited. And as I waited, I eyed row after row of glass bottles lined neatly and precisely along shelves that lined the wall from floor to ceiling. They contained many things, most of which I didn't recognise. There seemed to be various types and colours of bark-looking things, and various types of twig-looking things, and seeds and beans and many, many other types of things, I knew not what. On the other wall was a poster of a human body with all of the acupuncture points upon it and next to that was a poster showing many photographs. Each set of photos showed a before and after shot of someone with a partially bald head, and then a photo of the same person with much more hair than before. I was amazed, but incredibly sceptical. And in the corner of the room there was a large fridge, and in front of it was a long glass counter with a till upon it. Inside the counter were lots of different bottles and packets of all sizes and shapes, and they were unusual looking, as all of the writing on them were brush-stroked Chinese characters.

I was mesmerised, there was nothing in here that was at all familiar to me, and I hoped that amongst the unusual and exciting packets and bottles and twigs and bark that there was, hidden away somewhere, a cure for the bane of my life, my spots. Suddenly, as if by magic, the shopkeeper appeared behind the desk. She asked my name, in very broken English, and gestured, beckoning me to follow her into one of the little rooms at the back of the shop. I followed her past the colourful pictures of Chinese dragons, and into the little dark room. Inside the room sat a little Chinese woman, about fifty years of age, wearing a long white coat. She stood up and shook my hand gently, then gestured for me to sit. So I sat next to her on the small leather chair, in the half-light of the desk lamp. She asked me what was wrong and I pointed to my face full of spots. She closely examined them by twizzling her lamp around to shine directly into my face to interrogate the throbbing mass. Then I pointed to my legs, which had recently become covered in patches of red and angry eczema, like sprinklings of red ink onto a wet piece of tissue. I had been to the doctor about that too, stress related eczema apparently. He gave me some steroid cream for it, which seemed to make the eczema angrier and itchier, so I thought I'd get that looked at by the kind Chinese lady too. I felt a natural alternative to the steroid cream would be much better. She looked carefully at my legs, after the close inspection of my face, and scrawled something upon the record card she had made for me with my details on. I couldn't tell what she had written as that too was in Chinese. The tiny lady began to tell me I had too much yin, or was it yang, I can't remember, but I remember she said I had too much 'damp'. She then led me outside to the large counter full of pills and potions and picked up a little brown bottle and poured in a scoopful of spherical, chocolate brown, odd smelling dung balls, and told me to take five of them each day. It seemed like a huge dose to be taking, but she assured me that because they were herbal tablets they were not that strong, so to get an effect you had to take what seemed like a huge amount of them. Then she went to the fridge in the corner of the room and got out a little glass pot full of an ivory-coloured, orange-smelling cream. She told me to keep it in the fridge and put it on the eczema twice a day. And finally she reached up to one of the large glass jars from the shelves and poured out several large, white paper bagfuls of twig and bark-looking things. They looked as if someone had swept up the floor of a forest and put the leaf litter into the jar, and now she was pouring them out for me. I looked open mouthed at her – what on earth was I supposed to do with those? She told me to put one bag in to a saucepan with some water, bring it to the boil, and then simmer for fifteen minutes. Then once the liquid had cooled I was supposed to drink half of it on one day, and half of it the next day, and I had to repeat this scary proposition every couple of days. I was flabbergasted, but willing to try just about anything. When I got home I decided to make the twig tea straight away - no time like the present so they say. So I got one of my largest saucepans, put in one bag of the twigs, poured on some water, and let it boil then left it to simmer. When I went back in to the kitchen to turn the cooker off the most disgustingly pungent smell hit the back of my throat, a smell that I had never smelt the like of before, and I could feel my stomach begin to churn. I tentatively lifted the lid and as I did I recoiled in horror as the pungent pong slapped me in the face and I caught sight of the slightly soggy twig tump swimming in the putrid, blacky-brown, liquid bark bile. My lunch began to rise as I caught my breath. "My God, I've got to drink this!" I thought, horrified. Being foolishly brave, and desperate to give just about anything to help cure my spots a go, I got myself a mug. I carefully poured half of the rancid tarriness in to the mug, taking care not to pour any of the twigs and leaf litter in as well. I quickly put the lid back on the pan, so that the revolting smell wouldn't spread through the rest of the house, as the gloop would have to sit there until I finished it off the next day. I lifted the mug to my nose and had a small sniff. "Cor...Gee whizz!" I baulked with my eyes rolling. "How the hell am I going to drink this?" I put the mug on to the counter, got another mug and filled it with water, and got a ginger nut biscuit out of the cupboard, ready to take away what I knew was going to be a fantastically putrid taste. Okay, here goes!

I lifted the mug and glugged back the stinking tar, trying desperately not to breathe, as I knew that would make the taste worse. Then once I had taken my final glug, I shoved the whole ginger nut into my mouth and crunched it as fast as I could before I even took a breath. As I gasped my first breath, trying hard not to spit ginger nut across the kitchen units, the taste of liquid ashtray mingled with ginger nut, and hit my taste buds ferociously. And as it did I fought with the overwhelming urge to heave. I had never tasted anything quite as revolting as that before, and I haven't tasted anything as revolting as that since. It tasted as if I had boiled up manky, rotten, bin juice, and drunk it.

That is the only way I can describe how thick and black and utterly revolting it was.

But, despite the horrors of the twig tea, I continued to drink it as I had been instructed, and take the pills and rub the cream onto my legs. And month after month I would go back to the lady at the Chinese Health Centre, and each time we would try things a little differently, or try some different pills, but still it didn't rid me of the ghastly spots. The eczema on my legs improved, but my spots only improved slightly. So after months of trying I conceded defeat and begrudgingly went back to the doctor. I told him that I had really had enough of the spots and I really needed him to help me, I was nearly twenty-seven for goodness sake, I shouldn't look like this. After chatting to him for a while he said he was going to do a blood test to check that everything was okay, put me on a very strong contraceptive pill which would help to regulate my hormones he said, and told me to make an appointment for next week. So I went to the nurse, she took a blood sample, and off I went, a little bemused but much happier as at last someone was taking me seriously. The next week I went back to the doctor to get the results of my blood test. I sat in his big black chair and tried to read his face, as he opened my file and reacquainted himself with my notes.

"We've had your results back and it seems as if you have Poly Cystic Ovary Syndrome. I'd like to send you to the hospital to have an ultrasound to confirm this."

"Pardon me, Poly what?" I said confused.

"Poly Cystic Ovary Syndrome – it's caused by hormones not working as they should and therefore create cysts on the ovaries. The symptoms usually include heavy and very irregular periods, acne, facial hair, and problems with your weight. And you've had problems with your periods being irregular, and you've had problems with your spots," he explained.

"Well what does this mean?" I asked, feeling glad that at least I had found an explanation for my revolting complexion, but very anxious as to what the consequences of this might be.

"It's to do with some of your hormones not working properly, which makes you produce more testosterone, which in turn has caused your acne, and the cysts on your ovaries. The consequences of having PCOS, as it's called, is that it makes it quite difficult to conceive, and in some cases it causes women to become infertile. The contraceptive pill that I've prescribed should help regulate your hormones, which should improve your acne. The hospital will send you an appointment for the ultrasound scan."

Not only was my skin letting me down, but now my hearing was too.

"I'm sorry, could you say that again, because I thought you just said I might be infertile." I asked full of complete despair and disbelief. Surely he couldn't possibly have slipped something as important and devastating as that so flippantly into conversation.

"It is possible PCOS sometimes leaves women unable to conceive, and if they are able to conceive it usually takes a long time to succeed due to the damage that the cysts have caused and the fact that the times the eggs are released are so variable. Have you got any more questions you would like to ask?"

My head began to spin, "Er...No," I mumbled. "Thank you."

As I left the doctor's surgery my head began to spin even more and I felt dreadful. Infertile, infertile, infertile my head spat at me, and I began to feel incredibly sad and scared. 'I'll wait until I've had the ultrasound before I worry,' I thought, trying to convince myself that I would be all right.

The day of the ultrasound came, and I had done exactly as my instruction letter had said. I had drunk just over a pint of water (and a bit more for good measure), at least an hour (well two actually, just to be on the safe side) before I was due to have the scan, I didn't want to get there and it not work. I sat in the waiting room at the hospital with my mother. It was full of men and women of different ages and different races, all different, but all wearing the same worried faces. It smelt of that hospital smell that you don't get anywhere else, and was slightly too warm for comfort. The walls were all shabby, shades of pink and grey, unloved, and were covered with posters and information on all sorts of diseases and conditions. I tried to read some of them, but my eyes had begun to stream, and my concentration had left me as wave after wave of an overwhelming urge to wee took over. I think I had drunk a little too much liquid, a little bit too far in advance of the appointment, and now I writhed in belly-bursting agony as my body screamed "GO TO THE LOO!" But I couldn't, or they wouldn't be able to do the ultrasound, and to make matters worse the appointments were running slightly late. I was now wincing and fighting with myself as I stared at the toilet, over the top of my bloated belly, at the other side of the waiting room. It looked as if it was Heaven, and if they didn't hurry up I might well end up in Heaven, as I was about to explode and drench all of

140

the sad-looking people around me. And judging by their faces that would have really made their day for them! I began to chuckle at the ridiculousness of it all, which made my urges worse, and at last to my relief, in the non-weeing sense of the word, a nurse called my name. 'Thank God!' I thought as I waddled after her, trying hard not to wee all over the floor as I tentatively took each step. I lay terrified and taut on the slab as she put some clear jelly-type lotion on my tummy and began trying to scan my ovaries.

"I'm sorry," she said. I gasped, surely she wasn't going to ask me to drink some more water because she couldn't see my ovaries properly.

"I can't drink any more," I winced with tears in my eyes as she pushed on top of my over-full bladder with her instruments, "I'm going to wet myself."

"No," she laughed. "You're far too full for me to be able to see properly! Go and let some of it out!" I didn't need telling twice. I waddled out, in double time, and shot towards the toilet. I didn't even do up my trousers I was so desperate, so I don't know what the other patients must have thought as I shot past them, belly hanging out, and flies undone, and straight into the toilet. I have never known such relief as I felt at that precise moment, even though I was only allowed a 'tiny one'.

After I had composed myself I went back to the nurse and she continued with the ultrasound.

"Ah yes," she said as she pointed to the screen. "You definitely have PCOS as there are lots of cysts on your ovaries, see, you can see them here and here." She pointed to several areas on the screen. It all looked like grey splodges to me, but she must have known what she was looking at. She seemed quite cheerful as she pointed out these glorious cysts to me. 'It's not a bloody baby,' I thought to myself, 'I'm not pleased to see them, I don't want them there.' I was sure she was going to give me a photograph of them to show the proud father. I was devastated, totally devastated. After emptying the rest of my aching bladder I walked out into the car park with my aching heart, and holding my mother I broke down and cried. What had I done to deserve this? She hugged me warmly and reassuringly, but I knew deep inside that not only was I letting myself down, but I was letting her down. I knew all she wanted was to be a granny. I walked around in a daze for days. At school, I had to keep fighting back the tears, as little children constantly surrounded me; I felt gut wrenchingly sad that I may never be able to have one of my own. I saw the void that was my life panning out emptily in front of me. I would never feel the heart bursting joy of holding my own beautiful little baby in my arms, looking into their big blue eyes and smiling. Never having a child who looked to me for comfort and love and protection when they fell and grazed their knee, or needed my reassurance when they went bravely to their first day at school, or needed a special mummy's cuddle when the bogyman hid under their bed in the darkness at night. Never being able to be part of a 'proper' family. Never having anyone that would ever call me 'mummy'. Never being called mummy, ever. My heart was breaking. The emptiness and the devastation I felt was so overwhelming, I didn't know what I could do to take the pain away. I felt so sad and so lonely. I had never heard of Poly Cystic Ovary Syndrome before, and I didn't know who to turn to in order to express my fears, my sadness, and my sense of loss. I felt like I had been bereaved of a child that I had never had, and I felt a total sense of failure. So not knowing what to do and not knowing what to say, I turned to no-one, and I said nothing. I kept all of my fears, and my feelings, and my sadness, locked up deep inside me. I felt like a complete failure as a female, and I felt as if I wasn't a 'proper' woman. I felt asexual and dirty and empty and hopeless. As if something unique and totally precious had been stolen away from me and had left me with a hollow empty space where a baby should have been. What kind of pointless existence must it be to be put on this planet to procreate, and then be so utterly useless that you can't. Then I began to worry that no man would ever want me now, what use would I be if I couldn't provide children for him. I was pathetic and angry with myself, and I was angry with my own uselessness. And every time I looked into the mirror at my spots, they were a constant reminder of my failure as a real woman. I never spoke about it again with the doctor, as I could see no point, he had given me the pill and as far as he was concerned the conversation was over. So I pretended to the outside world that I was okay, and it didn't matter, and that I didn't really want any children anyway. But I lied, and inside, a part of me died.

I cried as I told Sylvia about my pain and my sense of loss, and my complete sense of failure as a fully functioning woman, and how totally and utterly devastated I had been. But then I continued to tell her about my new doctor, who I had been to see since I moved, and he had been far more upliftingly positive. He had told me that it was probably a lot of rubbish that

I wouldn't be able to conceive, and he took me off of the pill immediately. It was far too strong he told me, and was not actually helping to deal with the cause of the cysts. He put me on a tablet, which helps to regulate the insulin, which helps to regulate the hormones, which helps to reduce new cysts forming, or something like that. He filled me with new hope, and with the new hope came fewer and fewer spots, and I began to feel a little less self-conscious.

I chatted with Sylvia, and we looked at all of the new hope, and we tried to focus on that. I had to realise, yet again, that it was not my fault. I didn't do anything to cause the PCOS, it was just one of those things that happens, and I had to live with it as best I could, without the feeling of hopelessness, guilt, and failure as a woman. I had to convince myself that I wasn't hopeless, I was still a woman, no less of a woman than anyone else, and that there was still hope of maybe one day having a child of my own. I also knew I had to work at reminding myself that my skin was no longer quite so bad, and that even if I did get a spot or two, that didn't automatically turn me back into Frankenstein's monster. I had to begin to see myself as I was now, and not see myself as I was then. It's very easy to still see yourself as you were in the fattest, spottiest, ugliest part of your life, rather than seeing the truth staring back at you from the mirror. My self-image was appalling after Dean, my spots and my PCOS, so together we tried to think of ways of improving my self-confidence. I was still doing the exercise every day where I told myself that I loved me, and it was beginning to get easier to do. I was even able to look myself in the eye and do it, so we decided to carry on with that homework. Sylvia said that it didn't matter if I carried on doing that for the rest of my life, as it would keep me focused and remind me that I deserved love and that I was important.

I told Sylvia that I had made an effort to cleanse my room and give myself a clean new start in order for the cleanliness to seep inside me and begin to cleanse me too. And after thinking about it long and hard I told her that I had decided to try and make the same effort with myself. I was going to cleanse myself and give myself a fresh new start. The way I looked, the clothes I had, and the way I was all had to change and be new in order for me to start a fresh new life. Sylvia smiled and said that anything I did that I deemed to be valuable and positive was indeed a good thing to do. She walked over to the grey metallic filling cabinet in the corner of the room, rummaged through some files and brought back a piece of paper, this week's homework. And upon the piece of paper that she handed me were what looked like ten bubbles, each with a piece of positive advice written in them. I looked at the title, 'Positivity Vitamins'. I understood it then, they were little pills of self-esteem that you fed yourself when you were feeling low; a vitamin boost. Sylvia told me I had to choose one of the pills each day and read it out loud to myself throughout the day in order to give myself a boost. There were two that stood out to me, ' I realise I have nothing to prove, I do not rely on others, I am secure and confident in myself,' and 'I love myself, I cherish myself and I am doing the very best I know how in the circumstances I am in at any time'. I liked those; they struck a chord with me. She said that I might only relate to one of the 'pills', which was fine, and if I wanted to repeat the same self-esteem boosting vitamin every day then that was fine too. She also said that if I wanted to I could write my own pills and read them to myself, as long as they were constructive and totally positive.

"Okay," I smiled. " I'll give it a whirl." I was willing to give anything a whirl if it was going to help with my recovery. I said my good-byes and crunched my way down the gravel drive, homework and pebble in hand.

CHAPTER SIXTEEN

I opened my new rustic wardrobe door. I had bought it to go in my new room for my new beginning, along with a dressing table, a bookcase and a small table for doing my drawing and writing on. I had positioned the little table next to my window so that, while I was thinking and deliberating about the things I was going to write about or draw, I could gaze out across the rambling hills and meadows, and watch the large trees that swayed protectively beside the house. They were so close to my window that when I lay on my bed I could watch their branches rippling, seaweed like, as the tidal winds washed in and out, moving the leaves like sand. When the tide was calm the sand stayed still and glisteningly whispering, and when the tide was harsh and cruel it would wash the flotsam and jetsam from the sky and the tree tops, and leave a tide mark of deep debris washed and tangled around their roots and trunks. They were indeed beautiful and seemed to give out such a strong soothing energy. I couldn't say what it was but it was always there, I could feel it. I would watch them for hours and hours as they swayed and played and danced in the rain and the sun and the moonlight, as I lay there and thought and thought and thought. I thought about what my life had been, where I was now, and where I was going, and what indeed I was going to paint upon the nearly white canvas that was to be my new life. The trees helped me to focus as I watched them bend and sway and arch as they embraced the windy storms, and stand calm and peaceful in the sunshine, just rustling their leaves gently as the fairies flew quietly by. I wished I could be like them. And still I thought and thought and thought. And I would sit and watch the two enormous over-plump crows that jostled and tussled for prime position on top of the sagging telephone wire, which heaved and stretched and groaned under the enormous weight of the well-stuffed, clumsy birds. You could always hear them squawking and muttering and cursing each other, but they were never far from each other's side. They were just like brothers, fussing and fighting but always together. I used to chuckle at their antics, and I named them Ronnie and Reggie Crow, because they were big and dark and broodingly menacing, and would always bully and scatter the little birds which would come down onto the lawn to eat mother's stale crusts and cakes. And I would sit and watch them swaying on the telephone line for hours and hours, as they watched the world turn quietly by.

I spent a lot of time thinking and staring at the sky and watching, and as I did I would collect the little twinkles of thoughts or images or inspirations that floated past me. Thousands of twinkles, like particles of dust shimmering for one brief moment as they swirled and twirled their way through a sliver of sunlight cutting through the window. And each twinkly particle of inspiration that I had I would write down or draw into my dark forest green, hard-backed note pad. And the pictures and the ideas, all disjointed and unrelated, would spread across the page and make friends and dance together with other ideas. Sometimes the ideas were small and alone, and sometimes they gathered together like tumbling snowflakes and grew and rolled and grew and rolled into a whole snowball of inspiring ideas. Nothing was too silly or too childish to jot down, everything was valuable. And at night as I lay alone in the darkness, my subconscious creative mind would leak out and melt together with my conscious thoughts, spinningly twirl around and around together and flash pictures and phrases of exciting and unusual ideas. And I would thrash around clumsily with my net trying to catch these beautiful, rainbowy, flittering butterflies. But as soon as I turned the lights on, so that I could see to capture these elusive beauties, they were gone. And all I would be left with was a vague feeling that perhaps something most precious and valuable had passed me by, and was now lost for good. So I decided I needed to get a better net, one that would work in the dark, one that would capture these magically inspiring moments without damaging their delicate wings. And one day it came to me, I found a net, and that night I lay with it next to my head on the plumply puffed pillow. So as my thoughts jiggled and wiggled and merged with the dreams and fantasies of my subconscious mind I clicked 'record' on the small grey dictaphone. And there I lay, semiconscious in the darkness, with my eyes shut and my mind open; I would quietly share my night-time delights with myself, and beat away the demons. Then when the sun streamed into my room in the morning, and I felt awake and ready, I would rewind my night's recordings and play them back to myself, jotting down all of the things I could make sense of from the night-time ramblings. It was incredible to hear my mumbling, sleepy, dreamy voice twittering on and on, full of crazy ideas and mumbling expressions, and I found it really odd, as I could never remember saying any of the things that I listened to on the tape. It was like someone else had tiptoed in during the night and recorded many magical ideas for me. It was amazing as my day-time brain found it difficult to remember things, to express things and to come up with interesting and creative ideas, but my sleepy brain seemed to tap into a creative subconscious that still seemed to be functioning well and in a really inspiring way. So I used these thoughts and feelings and ideas to do bits and pieces of drawings and writing, which helped to fill the empty time I found myself with constructively, rather than filling it full of worry. I had always wanted to paint and write, and hopefully combine the two by writing and illustrating children's stories, and now I had a chance to toy with these ideas. It wasn't easy as my head was still clogged gloopily, was utterly thick and uncooperative, and after a small amount of concentration would send me to sleep to recuperate. But through the fuggy fog I saw small flashes of proper, clear, functioning thought, and I made the most of the little flickers that I had. Putting down my ideas on paper helped me to focus and helped me to have some point to my life, something to aim for, rather than focussing on the emptiness that spread out bleakly before me. It helped me to gently rekindle something that I loved which I had long ago buried and forgotten about. It was like I felt that I didn't deserve to do something that I was good at, I wasn't allowed to dream, to have goals, to have ambition. Dreams and aims in life were for other people, people with talent, people that were better than me. And now, very slowly, I was beginning to realise that no-one was better than me, as everyone was equal, and that I deserved these things too. So I decided that I was going to be positive, and if I was going to change my life and dare to dream, then I would have to try to do something for me and my own dreams, which I had denied myself for such a long time.

To do something that would make me happy. I had spent so much of my life trying to make other people happy, trying to fulfil their dreams, trying to do what I thought they wanted from me, trying to fulfil the goals that other people had set for me. Always trying to do what I thought other people saw as the 'right thing'. And by doing all of these things for everybody else but myself, I had managed to give myself a dream and happiness bypass. As long as I was making everyone else happy, I shouldn't be so selfish as to expect my own glimmer of happiness, or to be stupid enough to believe that I too could follow my dreams. So I took this time and space in my empty and confused life to dabble with my dreams, and to dip my toe tentatively into the warm, sparkling rock pool of happiness.

I looked inside the wardrobe, but could see nothing. Could see nothing but one pulsating, bulging pile of blackness. I reached into the gloom, and hanger by hanger, pulled the dark distant memories from the wardrobe and piled them onto a pyre on the floor. Each piece of what was once me looked sad and saggy and baggy, and was a variety of shades of black. My combat gear with battle scars. As I examined each one I saw photographs of sad times and I just wanted to tear them up. Tear up the album and throw them away. I didn't want reminding. I didn't want to keep being reminded of the things that I didn't want to see and the person that I didn't want to be. I didn't want to look at these photos any more; I wanted beautiful ones, fresh ones, sunny and colourful ones – ones that showed me smiling. I had had enough of this gloom. It all had to go. A clean start. A clean life. I wanted to see the new me, the phoenix, the me that I was going to become. I wanted the outside to convince the inside that I was going to get better, that I was going to change, that I was going to shine brightly again. I had spent too much time inside the cocoon and I wanted to prepare myself for when I was ready to hatch.

I had watched many times those TV shows where someone had nominated some sad, grey, flabby, shabby looking person to have a surprise hair, make-up and clothes makeover. And I would feel pangs of sadness and sympathy for the terrified person as they shuffled apologetically onto the stage, oozing embarrassment at themselves and feeling as if they didn't deserve this thing. They didn't even feel they deserved to be alive most of the time, and they certainly didn't believe that anyone could possibly make them look good and feel good. But once the makeover fairy had waved her magic wand the person would stride back onto the stage looking completely different, beautiful, together and glamorous. And they would be smiling and twinkling and would look happier than anyone had seen them in a long, long time. But most people didn't realise that the beauty only partially came from the makeup and the clothes and the hairstyles. It mostly came from a secret hidden place inside that person, which was unlocked by their new exterior, and made them feel good about themselves for the first time in a long while. And it was because of this that they oozed opulent confidence. It was themselves that had made them truly beautiful. It was themselves that had given out that radiant glow from their inner beauty, and they themselves had seen it for that brief moment in time, before they allowed themselves to fall back into the hole that they had briefly peeked over the top of. And I thought to myself, as I looked at the dirty black pile at my feet, 'If they can do it, then so can I!' But I didn't want to peek at it, I wanted to have it and I wanted to be it, all of the time.

So I got my mother to take me to a quiet country town where there were a few nice shops, as a few were all I knew I could manage, and I bought myself a new wardrobe of clothes, in baby blues, and lilacs and creams and even some things in pink. The colour that was far too pretty and girlie for someone as dirty and ugly as me to wear, but I fought with myself and I won. I even bought a selection of beautiful, white, delicate, lacy underwear, and a selection of new paints for the new face that I had discovered. And upon the new face I painted the new me. Inside I was still fighting with the blackness, with the demons, with the insecurities, and with the recurring nightmares of the past. But amongst all of this chaos there were flashes of light and beauty and hope, and these were the things that I chose to cling to, and I chose to continue to fight the rest. And with my new bright and colourful exterior came a new confidence, which came and went with my moods. And although it often went, at least it had come. And as time passed I came to realise that if I kept trying and trying and trying, no matter how many times my confidence would leave me, I was sure that it would keep coming back. And each time it came back it washed and left a little shiny smooth pebble glistening at my feet, which I would smilingly pick up and put with the others in the secret place where I kept them. And there they stayed, in the secret place, in the darkness, silently ready and patiently waiting for when I was ready to rebuild the dam.

CHAPTER SEVENTEEN

"You look really different today. Very pretty," smiled Sylvia encouragingly, as I sat curled up in the chair. And as I sat there, despite the pain that I felt inside, I felt just about ready give her the next instalment of the catalogue of nightmares that had put me here, made me ill, made me have to go to the counselling sessions.

I always took my job as a teacher very, very seriously and I always cared for the children's well-being and peace of mind as much as I cared about their education. So whenever someone was happy and laughing I would share their joyfulness with them, and whenever a child was sad or lonely or crying, I would take the time to see if I could help and see if they wanted to share their troubles with me. In my first year of teaching I had a little boy join my class. He was older than the others but he was put with me, as his level of ability was that of the children in the year group below his own. When the headmistress brought him to me on his first day in my class I saw before me, clinging to her hand so tightly that her fingers had turned white, a pale round-faced child, with his shirt-tails poking out from beneath his jumper. And he had a mass of curly dark hair and a frozen grin that screamed 'I'm terrified, please like me'. We made the wriggly scruffy little thing very welcome, and encouraged him to participate in all of the activities as a part of our class. He was a lovely little boy, but incredibly hard work. He found reading and writing quite hard and struggled desperately with them both, trying his best, trying to do things right, trying always to please. He was always the first to shoot his hand up enthusiastically to answer a question asked to the class, which he invariably gave the wrong answer to, but he was desperate, desperate to try. Desperate for approval, desperate for recognition, desperate for praise. And it was this desperation that always led him to be in the wrong place at the wrong time doing the wrong thing, which got him into lots and lots of trouble. He was often found to be doing something wholly inappropriate but which he considered to be helping me, or one of the other children, and he usually got things wrong in his desperate attempts to please. I spent hours and hours with him, trying to help him with all of the things that he found difficult, and he thought I was fantastic. He would come into the classroom and hand me a little card or a little model that he had made especially for me with his little pale face beaming from ear to ear, and when I smiled and thanked him for the little display of affection that he had handed to me, his face would light up like he had just won the greatest prize of all. And at break times when I was on duty he would come to me and ask to hold my hand. Then he would grab my hand with his mucky, snotty blue glove and gabble on to me inanely about all of the important issues in his six year old's world, all quick and nervous and smiley, as we walked around the playground. Sometimes I would tell him to go and have some fun and play with the others, and off he would run, helter-skelter with his shoelaces flapping. He would chase around madly after invisible things, as the wind blew wildly and tossed the rusty leaves around with him, and sometimes he played and talked with his friend who was not there. And sometimes he would play on the fringe of a group of the boys in his class, always looking over his shoulder to check to see if I was still watching him, always smiling. Always smiling but never happy. They would always let him join in, but he never seemed to fit in with them, or fit in anywhere at all. I suspected he didn't fit in at home either. His mother had the same dark curly hair and had the same dark shadows under her eyes. Her skin was pale, almost yellow, and she talked quietly but quickly in the same fast nervous way as Aaron. And every time I met her she could never hold my gaze, could never look me in the eye, and it would make me feel uneasy, as if something was terribly wrong. She would always listen to the suggestions that I made in order for her to try to help Aaron at home with his work. She seemed to try her best with him, but whatever she did always seemed to be crammed between all of the other things she had to do in her life, always busy, busy, busy. Aaron's stepfather was different. I could always hear him being stern and sharp with him, as if he was an irritating inconvenience, and whenever I tried to catch him to discuss the latest success or problem with Aaron he was no-where to be seen. He would shoot down the corridor like a red arrow, and Aaron would be trailing behind him, satchel and feet flying in the air like a kite. And if I wanted to speak to him I would have to sprint down the corridor after him in order to be able to catch up and have a chat. On the rare occasions that I caught a glimpse of the elusive man, and actually managed to catch up with him, he was always very disinterested and sharp. And no matter what came out of my mouth whether it was good or bad, he would always tell Aaron off. Never good enough you see, no matter what poor Aaron did. Always was wrong in his eyes. Occasionally I would have some wonderful news for him to pass on to his wife of some tremendous progress or some tremendous work, for which Aaron was burstingly proud of, and proud of the stickers and stars he had gained for his unexpected excellence. But his father would always dismiss it and pick up on a negative, something that was wrong, and Aaron's wide and nervous grin would melt off of his little pleading face and dribble into a puddle of sadness upon the floor at his feet, in front on his scruffy black scuffy shoes. And his head would hang low and his shoulders would sag as yet again he had been told he was a failure. He moved into the next class the next year and still his troubles continued. No matter what his teachers did, or what his teachers said, it made no difference. In fact the situation with his parents got worse. His mother was always close to tears and hysteria when she appeared, and his father very rarely showed his face. He would sit outside the school gates and toot the horn of his smart black sports car, and Aaron would go running like a startled chicken. Then one day his parents decided that they couldn't be bothered to pick him up at all, so at the age of seven he had to catch the school coach all on his own. The coach didn't leave until 5.00pm, when the senior school had finished, and one of the older girls would come down and collect Aaron to go on the coach. And while he waited for five o'clock to arrive he would wander up and down the lonely corridor waiting, with his little blazer on and his satchel in his hand. Often, as I sat in the peaceful stillness of the classroom at the end of the day, filling in records, marking work and writing plans ready for the next day, I would see a little mop of dark hair and two pleading eyes peep around the corner of the classroom door. And with desperation in his voice he would ask me if there was anything that he could help me with or if there were any jobs for him to do. I always found something for him to help me with, so that he felt needed and wanted and proud of the help he had given, and he would go off to find his senior school carer with a little bit more of a spring in his step than when he had arrived in my room. And occasionally, first thing in the morning, he would come and find me in my classroom to give me something he had made for me at home the night before. He was an adorable little boy, but he always seemed to radiate sadness, no matter how wide his grin was.

That summer Guy and I were decorating the whole of his house before we moved his furniture back in, which was at my house. The sun blazed in through the windows as I rollered the lemony yellow paint onto the once peach walls of the bedroom. It was hot and sticky, and I was admiring the splattering of yellow custardy spots on my arms and on my legs where my shorts had ended, when the phone rang. I ran down the stairs to answer it. It was my mother.

"I've just been reading the evening paper and there's an article in there about a little boy from your school who was found washed up dead on the beach where he was on holiday in France. They say he must have drowned while he was playing on the beach."

"That's awful," I gasped, horrified. "Who was it?" I held my breath, not really wanting to know what the answer was.

"Ah, hang on, let me look...It was Aaron Lewis, and he was eight. Do you know him?" she asked, her voice full of worry.

I wracked my brain, well I knew Aaron Lewis, but it couldn't be him, he was only seven. Then my stunned and mortified brain pushed forward the fact that he was indeed eight, but he had been kept back a year which made me think he was younger than he was. My head froze in stunned horror, how could someone so young, so innocent, with such a kind heart, be gone, be dead, be no more? It couldn't be real, it just couldn't be. I slid down the wall and sat in a pile of collapsed and dumbstruck disbelief. 'It can't be true, it can't be true, it has to be a mistake, an awful and cruel mistake,' I thought as I placed the receiver back onto the phone base. I sat on the floor, numb, dumbfounded and suspended in total and utter shock. I couldn't believe it; it wasn't true.

The phone began its violent ring again, which made me jump from the frozen puddle on the floor. And the voice at the other end was a teaching colleague confirming the sad and horrible truth.

"I'm so, so sorry," the voice said sadly. "Are you alright my love?"

"I'll be fine..." I whispered through the tears as I put the phone back down.

I went back upstairs and picked up the custardy roller and carried on painting. The sun was still shining and I was still painting, and it seemed as if it was a hallucination, a horrible black dream. The roller went up and down all by itself as I shook with sadness and horror at the thought of the poor little mite alone, drowning in the cruel, cool sea. My imagination fired morbid pictures of what had happened, and I fought with them through the tears as my body trembled with anger. Where the hell had his parents been and why the hell didn't anyone see him or save him? And as my head span in fiery anger the roller carried on up and down and up and down as if nothing had happened, but my tears betrayed me. Guy came in and looked at my tear stained face.

"What have you done?" he barked, thinking I had mucked up the painting or spilt the paint or done something wrong as he always thought I did. I filled him in with the sad, sad tale as the tears poured and poured and the sadness was unbearable. I had become so close to him, as you do with all of the children that you teach. You spend five days a week with them for a year, and in that year you probably spend more time with the children than many of their parents did, so you couldn't help but become close to them.

"That's a shame," he said unemotionally as he walked away to put some lager in the fridge. "I've invited the neighbours around for a beer in a minute."

"Can we just go home, my head's thumping really badly Guy, I feel terrible.." I sobbed. The paint fumes, the heat and the terrible sadness were all taking their toll and I felt really, really awful.

"Look, I've invited them now, so if you don't feel well just stay here and lay down. We'll go home later."

"They won't mind," I pleaded; we were always spending time with them, it wasn't a special occasion or anything, just him trying to be liked, trying to be the centre of attention.

"No way are we going home! I've invited them for a beer and I'm not letting them down, so you'll just have to lay down here until I'm ready to go back to yours." And off he stormed leaving me curled up on the floor of the bedroom. I couldn't argue, it never got me anywhere, and my head was about to tear in two as it was throbbing so much. The sadness I felt deep inside was utterly overwhelming and completely consuming.

I could hear him below the open bedroom window, laughing and joking with a couple of the neighbours in the garden, and making out like I didn't exist as I lay on the floor of the bedroom. And as I lay there I kept trying to keep myself calm, trying not to let my tears tumble, as the more upset I got the more my head throbbed, and the more my head throbbed the more upset and scared I got. So I tried to keep a grip on the shreds of calm that I had, and I lay and quietly watched the evening sun's rays move gently across the newly painted wall, until they were eventually replaced by the darkness, and I could no longer see the colour of the paint. As the conversation flowed, along with the beer, I heard one of them ask where I was, as they had all assumed I was not there. He explained what had happened and I could hear disbelief in their voices as they asked him why he wasn't looking after me, making sure I was okay, and why he hadn't been up to check up on me for the whole of the time that they had been there. And I held my breath as I waited for the reply and when it came I wasn't surprised.

"She'll be fine."

I closed my eyes and tears rolled silently down my cheeks, so much love, so much comfort, so much support, always there when I needed him most.

I heard footsteps on the stairs, the door swung open, and Clive came in. He put the light on, and the sharp brightness made my salty eyes squint and sting, and then he crouched down next to me and sat on the floor. He had come to see how I was and comfort me since Guy wasn't interested when he had friends to entertain. It was more important for him to impress his friends than it was for him to be there when I needed him most. After spending ten minutes talking to me Clive told me he was going to get everyone to leave so that Guy could take me home, and he kissed my hand gently and went back downstairs and out into the back garden. I could hear chatting and voices and after about five minutes the three neighbours had left. Guy thundered up the stairs and burst into the bedroom.

"Come on then, let's bloody well go back to yours," he shouted angrily, and I could tell by his face and from the smell of his beery breath that he was really drunk. I pleaded with him for us to get a taxi, but he just shouted and swore and said that if I wanted him to take me home then he would bloody well take me home! I told him to stay, and go and have a drink with the neighbours, and I would get a taxi back on my own. But he was mad, mad, mad and bundled me into the car, despite my protestations; and I was too weak, grief stricken and in pain to fight him. If we crashed because he was drunk then we just crashed; by this time I just didn't care any more. So he swerved his way dangerously back to my house the long way through the dark country lanes, so that no-one would see him and he wouldn't get stopped by the police. When we got home he ranted and raved about this and that and a lot of indecipherable nonsense, then collapsed in the armchair and fell asleep. I crawled into bed, on my own, with my throbbing head and my breaking heart, curled myself into a little black ball and cried myself to sleep.

The day of the funeral was terrible. The sky was black and thunderous and I was dreading it. Funerals were dreadful enough when it was expected or when it was someone old, but to have to go to the funeral of a child was unbearable. Especially when it shouldn't have happened. I had found out that his parents had been at the bar on the beach when he had gone missing. They thought he would be okay on the beach playing, they said he could swim and would be safe because the lifeguards were watching him and they had an eye on him too. Eye on him my foot! How could you keep an eye on him from the bar? They thought he would be okay. But he was not okay was he? And I knew he couldn't swim, he had turned down a pool party invitation from one of his classmates because he couldn't swim, and it was obvious too that the life guards were not there looking after him, it wasn't their job to look after him. His parents though should have been. I knew they didn't care for him, I knew they saw him as an inconvenience, and I was so, so ragingly red hot angry at them as this should never have happened. I felt in my aching heart that I, and his other teachers, had shown him more love, and cared more for him, than his parents ever had, and I was very angry.

I sat there, on the bottom-aching wooden pew, in the small, dark, cold church, with Aaron's class teacher and the headmistress. I felt insignificant and alone even though the church was full to bursting with people of all ages, who had all come to say good-bye to the little ray of sunshine that was Aaron. And as the sad, slow, raw, strains of the organ began I caught sight of the small, white, boy-sized coffin with silvery handles, and upon the coffin was a yellow teddy bear and a big red car both of which were made of flowers. Aaron had loved cars, he had often drawn them on the cards that he had made for me, and my eyes began to quietly weep. The small white coffin was carried in by Aaron's stepfather, and three men I did not recognise. His stepfather's face was blank and cold, like a non-feeling shark, as he walked slowly along the cold stone aisle. And following the coffin was his grief stricken wailing mother whose legs were collapsing under her with sadness; she was being held up by her mother and her daughter, one under each weak and trembling arm. My head was screaming, "Fraud! Fraud! Fraud!" as she wept and she wailed. And I thought, if she had really loved him that much she would never have left him alone on the beach to play and to drown, drown, drown. My anger seethed. There were other relatives who followed behind the coffin, all of them finding it dreadfully difficult to stop themselves from bursting out with tearful grief, and I wondered if they knew the truth, if they felt like me. The service was difficult, and I found it impossible to continue to hide behind my professional mask, so my human face began to crack through. When we began to sing his favourite hymn my grief burst through the cracks and drenched me, leaving a sea of tears washing around my feet. I could never understand why hymns were sung at funerals as they were the point at which people who had been managing to hold things together finally burst out in inconsolable tears and grief. I tried so hard to keep my tears inside, and each time one escaped and trickled down my cheek I caught it in my handkerchief, which by now was despairingly damp. I glanced sideways and watched the tears of his class teacher tumbling down her face, which gave me permission to release mine, and they washed out in torrents. The headmistresses face was as stony as the graves and totally unemotional. If she had a heart, which was debatable, it was made of solid granite. And as the hymns carried on I became angry with God too. All these songs about how loving and forgiving He was and how He made the world a glorious place to be, well I could see no glory. I could see neither glory nor happiness from this particular action that He had taken. I could see no rhyme or reason or point to the whole damn thing. Yes, I was angry with God too. And I didn't care if He knew it.

When the heart-wrenching service was over, we watched as Aaron was slowly carried away to be buried. His close family followed behind him, and it felt like my heart went with them. I tried to regain my composure as I made my way out of the church with the others, and tried desperately to keep it as I walked through the huddles of parents of the other children in his class, all of whom held each other and sobbed for the loss of someone so young and so innocent. The little light in the darkness. I kept together behind my mask of professionalism alongside his class teacher, who also hid well behind her mask, and we both stared angrily at the granite woman who had not shed one tear during the whole of the most excruciatingly moving and sad funeral that either of us had ever been to. I hated her. Hated her with a passion. As we walked out into the grey drizzle my colleague suggested that we went for a drink in the pub next to the church. We both needed to calm down and compose ourselves before we went back to school to teach, but the woman with the barbed wire around her heart said no. We had to get back to our classrooms and teach, and we had to carry on as if nothing had happened. I had always known she was a poisonous hard bitch, but I had never quite appreciated as to what extent. Today my opinion of her had sunk even lower than a snake's slithering belly. I would never forget that lovely but lonely sad little boy, and I would never forget the anger that I felt towards his parents, and the anger towards myself at not being able to have changed the way that his parents didn't love him. I had loved him though, that sad little boy with the desperate grin, and I held on to that thought, held it deep in my heart as I read the words in the card that I had kept from him. 'To Miss Williams, I love you...' and through my tears I'd smile.

I talked all of this through with Sylvia, and the thing I felt most was anger; red hot, volcanic anger – anger towards his parents, anger toward myself, and anger about the unfairness of it all. We talked and talked and I began to realise that anger was a completely normal response to such a tragic event. And when I thought sensibly about it I shouldn't have been angry at his parents. I'm sure they loved him in their own way, and I was sure that they couldn't possibly have wanted this to happen. They must have been heartbroken, and indeed feeling extreme guilt and hopelessness. I also shouldn't have been angry with myself. I had given him much love and support and done all that I could have possibly done to make him a success in the eyes of his parents. I had tried, and he had thought the world of me. I had made him feel good about himself, made him proud of himself, and made him smile. I couldn't have done anything different, I couldn't have made this tragedy not happen. I shouldn't have been angry at myself, I shouldn't have felt guilty, and I shouldn't have felt like I should have done more. I couldn't have done more. I was also told that it was common for people to feel angry about someone being taken away from them so tragically, it was just one aspect of the grieving process that many people go through. It felt good to release some of the anger; it was good to release the unfounded feelings of blame. I felt so much lighter as I began to let it all go, and as I did I began to remember the happy times that I had shared with the little grinning boy.

But that was not the only trauma that I had to deal with that year; there had been upset after upset and sadness after sadness. And each traumatic event and upset that took place drained me of more and more of my emotions. And as I was dragged down and down by the upsets and the pain, to my horror all of the nightmares from my past danced out of the closet and joined in with the devilish fun. And as my emotional reservoir drained to a tiny puddle I found that I wasn't able to react in a normal emotional way to the events that took place, day after day, as I had nothing left to react with. Pain became my normal reality, and as time went by I forgot that any other feeling but pain existed. I found myself becoming more and more numb as I drowned in the river of pain, and the events that took place which would normally be devastating didn't affect me any more, they just made the river swell and the lead in my legs become heavier, and I would just carry on swimming. Until one day the last drop of pain dripped into my river, after months and months and months, and my head dipped under the dark, heaving, tumbling currents and finally I drowned.

Four months after Aaron had died my great-grandmother was taken into hospital quite suddenly. Although she was eighty-nine she was fighting fit and a fine picture of health. She always put on her eye shadow and blusher and lipstick, was always well dressed, and never went anywhere without putting on her earrings and necklace and silk scarf. She was the head of the family and everyone looked up to her and went to her for advice when life went wrong. She was always bright and alert, with a mischievous twinkle of life in her eyes, as she told us all off and kept us all in order. Then one day, just after Christmas, she suddenly had trouble breathing and felt kind of funny, so she went into hospital. After many tests they told us that it was a problem with her heart, and that it was dangerously weak. Everyone was distressed and everyone was upset, especially my mother. She had a very, very close relationship with Nanny Joan, and whenever she was troubled it was her that she turned to. She loved Nanny Joan a great deal.

Mum came around to pick me up to go and visit her. I already felt terrible. Things were going dreadfully wrong with Guy, and I had begun to turn to my friend, the bottle. When mum came to get me I had already had a couple of glasses of wine, to numb the pain from Guy and to numb the pain of life. I knew that I shouldn't, but I couldn't cope without it.

We walked along the dark walkway from the car park, the winter light had begun to fade and dark shadows began to disguise the shabbiness of the hospital walls and the curling paint on the windows. We stepped into the florescent brightness of the corridor, and along with the stinging brightness of the unnatural light came the stinging reality that I was about to see my great-grandmother, and she was very, very ill. The glasses of wine had made everything seem harsher and brighter, and apprehension grasped my insides tightly. I had to keep smiling though as my mother was dreadfully upset. We pushed open the door to my great-grandmother's ward and walked slowly past each neatly and tidily tucked-in bed. And in each crease-free bed sat a crumpled and withered old lady, looking sad or confused or mumbling and grumbling to herself. Some of them lay and slept and loudly snored like a row of wrinkly grey elephants with colds. And as I looked at them I couldn't decide which flowers had wilted the most, the pots of multicoloured flowers that were dotted here and there, or the flowers that sat droopily in each bed. The old ladies all looked so saggy, so fragile and so, so scared. They must have all been sat there wondering if they were ever going to go home again, and were reminiscing and looking back at their sad, flat lives. And I wondered if they sat there full of regrets and if onlys, and were all wondering, 'did I do all that I wanted, did I achieve my goals, am I happy with how things turned out, am I happy with my lot?' I suspected from the sadness in their eyes and their radiating discontent that they were indeed disappointed. Disappointed with themselves, disappointed with their lives, disappointed with everything. As I walked past the Ethels and the Ediths and the Lillians and the Ednas I thought, and I hoped, that when I got to their ages, and if I was sitting there looking back at my life, that I would be smiling because I had achieved all I had wanted, seen all I had wanted, and I had been exactly who I had wanted to be. And I hoped that I would be content with the way that my whole life had turned out. But who the hell was I kidding. I could see my future, and could see my face etched on to the unhappy Ethels, all sad and lonely and dreadfully disappointed with the mess that was my life. And there I would sit, about to shuffle off this mortal coil, unfulfilled, unhappy, unloved. I was already drinking to cope, and my life was already a complete disaster. My mother stopped at the foot of the bed of a lifeless, limp, grey old lady who looked as if someone had deflated her and left her sagging at the top of the bed. Her eyes spoke of contentment, but the twinkle had been dampened, and the light in her eyes was shadowy and dull. I couldn't work out why mum had stopped, who was this she was talking to? I looked on the wall beside her head for her name, and there it was in big blue felt pen, 'Joan Jones', my great-grandmother. I gulped with shock; someone had stolen Nanny Joan and replaced her with a deflated grey balloon. But it was true, it was her, it was really happening. My mum and the rest of the family tried to chivvy her along, cheer her up and make light of the harrowing situation. We all pretended everything would be okay, and we all looked into each other's eyes and knew that we were lying. Nanny Joan may have been fading, but her mind was still as sharp as a tack. When the others went off to get a cup of tea she held my mum gently by the arm and pulled her slowly down close to her face. She looked deep into my mother's eyes,

"This is it, isn't it Jewel?" she asked quietly, searching my mothers face for the answer. My mother need not have replied because despite the smile on her face her eyes bled with the truth. "Don't be so daft, you'll be fine. You'll be out of here in no time." Nanny Joan laid her head back gently onto the pillow and smiled knowingly as she held my mothers hand. She always knew everything.

The next day my mum phoned to say she was coming to pick me up to go in to see my great-grandmother again. This time I was determined, no matter how bad things were, that I would not have a drink before I went. I had felt really bad about the previous day, even though I was sure no-one knew. I felt really, really guilty, no matter how bad my life was I shouldn't have stooped to that. As I sat there in the lounge, with my coat on ready to go, the phone went again, but this time it was my father, and he wasn't the bearer of good news. He had been phoned and told that Nanny Joan had just died, and he told me that I had to stop mum from going to the hospital, as there was nothing she could do. My heart went cold, not only had I just been told that my great-grandmother had died, but I had to break the news to my mother, and I knew she was going to be totally devastated. I asked Guy if he would take himself and his son to the neighbours' house so that I could tell mum on her own without an audience. So off they went, and I sat there, trying desperately to hold the tears inside so that I could be big and brave and be there for my mother, to comfort her and care for her, as I knew she would fall apart. In my mind I went over and over and over what I was going to say to her, so that it all came out right, and so that I didn't say the wrong thing or say something that might make it worse. I didn't know quite what would make it worse, but I didn't want to do it nonetheless. I still had my coat on when she arrived, as I was cold and numb and unable to think straight, let alone think about taking my coat off.

"Come on in, sit down," I said with a crooked smile that gave away my news. She sat down quietly on the sofa and looked up into my face with a sad and knowing expression upon hers.

"I'm really, really sorry mum but I've just had a phone call from dad to say that Nanny Joan has died."

She looked into my face as the saddest of all sad news sunk into her head and into her heart. She began to sob and sob and floods of tears emptied down her flushed and burning cheeks. I held on tightly to my emotions as I held her tightly. I had to be strong, I had to be strong. I did my best to comfort her, and offered her a 'nice cup of tea', like you should do in a proper English crisis, but she declined as she wanted to go straight home. She never felt comfortable in Guy's company and I was sure she didn't want him seeing her like this.

"Do you want to come with me? Will you be alright?" she asked through her streaming tears of sadness.

"I'll be fine," I lied, as she got into the car and drove away. And as I saw her disappear down the street my knees buckled and my sorrow roared forth like a sad and angry lion. I was crying for my mum, I was crying for my great-grandmother, I was crying for myself, I was crying for every sad thing that was happening inside and all around me. I phoned up Clive and told him Guy and Steven could come back now as mum had gone. Clive said he was so sorry to hear the news and would tell Guy. Two hours later Guy rolled in with Steven. Steven ran in and sat beside me, put his little hand on my knee and looked into my eyes.

"Are you alright?" he asked with concern in his voice. "I know you must be very sad as my granddad died and I was very sad too. You'll be okay, I'm okay now, I'm not sad any more." He smiled encouragingly at me and ran off to play his computer games. Guy said nothing. I sat on the sofa and cried, and still Guy said nothing. I made myself a drink and sat on the chair as Guy and Steven rolled around laughing at something on the television, and still he said nothing. He blanked me completely, like I didn't exist, like I just wasn't there, and inside my heart was breaking. All I needed was a hug, all I needed was a kind word or a smile or an "it'll be okay," but nothing. I just wasn't there. I couldn't stand it any more, I walked out of the back door and down the lane to Dave's house, Guy's best friend, who was rapidly becoming my best friend and ally. I went in through his back door, as we always did, and broke down into inconsolable sobbing. He opened a bottle of wine and after placing a large glass of red into my hand gave me a huge and comforting hug. He said he couldn't believe that Guy was such an uncaring and thoughtless bastard and that he certainly didn't deserve me.

"Look, I'm going to the pub soon, why don't you come with me and let the bastard get on with it on his own." I smiled but I knew I couldn't go, he was obviously mad enough with me already, and I certainly didn't want to make a bad situation worse. Dave tried and tried to make me go, but I knew I couldn't. I just couldn't. A little knock sounded at the back door, and Steven came in,

"Daddy says you've got to come home," he said, delivering the message perfectly. Dave looked at me and shook his head.

"I've got to go," I said with puffed up eyes, as I hugged Dave and thanked him for being there for me yet again, and out into the darkness I went. When I got back he still wasn't speaking to me, and for the life of me I couldn't figure out why. That night I lay alone in bed, Guy had decided to sleep in with Steven, and in the darkness tears streamed down my cheeks and soaked silently into my pillow – tears for the loss of my great-grandmother and tears for the loss of my life that was falling apart and crumbling all around me.

I know we should come to expect the deaths of our nearest and dearest when they are old and frail and unable to care for themselves, but Nanny Joan was nothing like that. She was alive and vital and the rock of the family, and naively we all thought that she would live forever. So even though she was very old we were all really shocked and really upset and really surprised. And I felt so, so guilty that the last time that I ever saw her I had been drinking, and I hoped that if she was looking down from Heaven then she would see the mess that was my life and understand and forgive me. Sylvia smiled and said that she was sure that she would forgive me, and that I should forgive myself too. She said it was normal to feel guilt when someone died, guilty about the things that you did or didn't do, and guilty about the things that you did or didn't say. It was a pot of knotted guilt spaghetti, difficult to untangle and very hard to swallow. And once you realised this and that it was normal to feel these things, then you should just forgive yourself and let it go. I felt a little lighter after we had talked about it and I tried to alleviate some of the guilt that had been eating away at me for months and months. We talked about Guy's reaction and I told her that he had said to me the next day that he didn't like talking about death, so that's why he didn't want to talk to me. I could understand that maybe he found it difficult, but I was so, so mad and disappointed because if he had really loved me he would have overcome his own feelings, and been there for me to comfort me and been there when I needed him the most. But he had let me down. Let me down really, really badly. He always found an excuse for everything, and everything was always my fault, he was good at making everything turn out to be my fault. And I hated him. Hated him with a passion. But that was next week's session.

"I can see that Guy is still inside your head most of the time, am I right?" Sylvia asked, already knowing the answer. And she was right – as always. He was always there, eating away at me, making me feel sad and bad and downright stupid. There were so many 'Whys' that I just needed answering, and so many things that I just didn't understand, that sometimes it felt like my head would explode with the man that had pressed my button of destruction. I hated it and I hated him and I didn't want him in there any more. I didn't want to hear his voice, I didn't want to hear his name, and I didn't want to see his face. I just wanted it to disappear, to go away for good, forever, so that I could get on with my life and rebuild it bit, by bit.

"He's always there inside my head. I can always see him and I can always hear him and I just want him to go away," I said with my head in my hands, full of despair.

"Right then!" said Sylvia getting up out of her chair. "Get up!"

So I did, as I knew it was always best to do what she told me as usually the things that she told me to do would eventually make me feel much, much better.

"Now then," she said, "I want you to stamp your feet up and down as hard as you can like this," and she stamped up and down as hard as she could, marching around the room like someone trying to put out a carpet which was on fire. "And I want you to shout and scream, at the top of your voice, as loud as you can, 'GET OUT OF MY HEAD! GET OUT OF MY HEAD! GET OUT OF MY HEAD!' And I want you to keep stamping and keep screaming until you feel like he has finally gone from your head."

'My God she's finally flipped!' I thought. But I did as I was told. And at first my stamping was half-hearted and quiet, and my shouting was weak and positively pathetic. But as I allowed myself to stamp harder and harder, and I allowed myself to scream louder and louder, I began to feel better and better. So I got louder and louder and stamped harder and harder until the whole room shook with my screams and the floor bounced underneath my angry, heavy, battering feet.

"GET OUT OF MY HEAD! GET OUT OF MY HEAD! GET OUT OF MY HEAD!" I screamed and shouted and roared with all of my might and all of my strength until tears poured from my eyes. Tears of anger, tears of hate, tears of frustration, tears of disappointment and tears of sadness for the way things turned out. And then the anger and the frustration began to ebb away, and finally he disappeared, and I collapsed back into the chair and wiped away the tears with my sleeve, and I laughed and laughed as my head was clear for that moment in time, and I felt a whole lot better.

"Feel better now?" asked Sylvia smiling. "That will have woken them up downstairs, I think they were in a meeting actually! Oh well never mind! You should do that any time you feel like it! Do it at home, do it in the garden, go to the top of a hill and do it! Just do it till it makes you feel better!" she smiled. And I smiled back.

"That feels much better!" I grinned.

Then Sylvia gave me this week's homework, which I found to be rather appropriate. I had to write a letter to Guy and tell him all of the things that I hated him for, and all of the things he had done that had made me feel bad, and all of the hurt and the pain and the anger. No holds barred. 'Did I have enough paper to write all of it down?' I thought. She also asked me to bring some photos of him, I didn't know what for but I trusted her. She had helped me a lot so far.

She asked me how I felt now and what else I could do that might lift my spirits further, might make me feel better, might carry on helping me dig myself out of the big black hole.

"I feel as if my spirit is broken, like my soul is smashed to bits," I said. "I know that sounds silly."

"It doesn't sound silly at all," Sylvia smiled, with her inner calm glowing and radiating out into the room. "If it's your spirit that needs healing then you should go and have it healed," she said completely rationally, like it was the most sensible and logical thing to do in the whole world.

"Find a spiritual healer in the phone book, they can usually be found at natural healing centres, and go heal your spirit," she said. Of course! Why didn't I think of that! It's so obvious! She had a way of making abnormal things seem like the most normal and ordinary things to do. Of course, that's what everyone does; they go to a spiritual healer! I wasn't so sure. But I thought about this as I went on my way, feeling flat and drained like an empty fish pond, and I was the gasping, flapping fish left at the bottom, trying desperately to breathe, to stay alive, to survive. Talking about my troubles took so much out of me.

I thought long and hard about what she said and I thought to myself that I had once believed in the power of the mind, and in the more spiritual and magical side of life, so I decided to give it a go and be brave. I had done many things that I had never done before in order to try and make myself better, so I thought I might just give this a go too.

CHAPTER EIGHTEEN

I walked up and down and up and down the streets of the town centre looking desperately for the Natural Therapy Centre. I looked at every plaque on every wall and every sign above every shop, but still I couldn't find it. I was starting to panic as if I didn't find it soon I was going to be late. And I really didn't want to be late as I was already perspiring with nervousness as well as the hiking I was doing around the hilly streets. In desperation I retraced my steps back to the steep car park where I had parked the car, and thought I'd try and follow the garbled directions once more to see where I had indeed gone wrong. 'Now then, steps at the corner of the car park, let me see,' I thought as I stood and surveyed the meandering maze, spider webbing its way down the hill in front of me. And then I spotted some steps at the corner of the car park, a small, awkward, uneven set of steps, and not the steps that I had originally taken.

'You total buffoon!' I thought as I tiptoed down the old stone staircase and onto the winding, sloping side street. And then, right in front of me, I noticed a plaque on the wall, 'Natural Therapy Centre - Up steps and second black door on the left.' I looked up above me, and there was a high grey stone wall with painted black railings on the top. And behind the railings seemed to be a garden, as bits and pieces of it were hanging and dangling raggedly between the rails and trailing down the side of the high stone wall. Cut into the wall was a set of steep stone steps that I climbed tentatively and found myself on a path that went through the two small front gardens of two tall and old-looking, grey houses.

The gardens looked slightly scruffy but cared-for all the same, as if someone did love them, but never quite seemed to have enough time to tend them properly. I walked along the cracked concrete path, past the first yellow front door, and entered through the heavy black door with the shiny gold plaque, 'Natural Therapy Centre' it said. I swallowed my nervousness as I entered into this new and strange environment, my mouth was dry and my forehead clammy as this was all so alien to me. An older lady, in her sixties, with thick glasses, a tangerine mohair jumper, lovely matching slacks and a head full of tight grey curls indicated to me to take a seat with a variety of gesticulations as she tried to answer the caller on the other end of the phone and deal with me all at the same time. I took a seat and looked at my feet in the tiny, sparsely decorated waiting room. What on earth was I doing? I thought to myself. I felt like running out, like running and running and running away, but I didn't want to look completely foolish, and I didn't want to pooh-pooh it and disregard it without giving it at least one try. No, I was going to go through with it, come what may; and I was going to keep a very, very open mind about the whole thing. 'Mind over matter, that's the key,' I thought. My rambling thoughts were broken by the receptionist, who had now finished her phone call and was asking who I was and who I had an appointment with.

"I'm Rachael Williams, and I've got an appointment with Rosa Grey," I squeaked out to the now calm lady with the odd looking owl-like eyes, who was assessing me from behind her untidy, disorganised desk.

"Lovely!" she said and I heard a buzzer announce my arrival in one of the rooms down the dark twisting corridor. A door opened from halfway along the corridor, and a wise-looking lady with a flowing purple skirt and frilly white blouse floated down the corridor like a spectre, with her long grey hair fluttering behind her as if caught by some unexpected breeze. She smiled at me and asked me to follow her – which I did – down the dark, narrow corridor with the yellow linoleum tiled floor, and into the tiny room from which she had first appeared.

"Sit down," she said, pointing at an orange plastic chair. The room was small, eerily quiet, and again sparsely decorated with plain cream walls. And in the centre of the small room was a large, flat, black leather platform-type bed, the sort of thing you might imagine a leather clad operating table to look like. I felt very uneasy, and suddenly very foolish, as I didn't know exactly what I was going to say to her.

"Right let us begin, what have you come to see me about and what is it you want me to do for you?" She seemed a little abrupt. Or maybe she wasn't abrupt at all, maybe it was just my imagination, or maybe it was just my nervousness and embarrassment as I wasn't quite sure how to articulate what my problem was, and I was sure she could already see inside my head and see that I was one big fool. But I tried my very best to explain that I had been suffering very badly from depression and that I felt like I needed my spirit healing, and as the words fell clumsily out I was sure she was going to turn me away as I sounded so utterly foolish. But instead of turning me away her face softened and she began to explain what she did and what she was going to do with me today. She told me that her main job was lecturing about spirituality, and the classes that she taught about spirituality had taken off in a very big way and were very well received, which she seemed extremely pleased about. But as well as this, once a month, she came to the Natural Therapy Centre to help people in need of healing, people like me. I was surprised, as she seemed so together and extremely academic, not at all woolly-headed as I had imagined she might be. She explained to me what she was going to do and it seemed so straightforward, so simple, almost like an exact science, which I suppose to her it was. So I took off my shoes and climbed trustingly on to the black leather bed and lay down. With the flick of a switch the bed whirred up to the level of her hips and stopped. 'Relax, relax, relax,' I told myself, 'it will be alright, nothing bad is going to happen to you.'

"Now then, close your eyes," she instructed, and I did as I was told and closed them tightly and continued to listen very, very carefully.

"I am going to take you on a journey, and the journey will take you wherever you want to go as the journey is in your imagination. But I will help you and guide you on your way. When I tell you to imagine something, you do it, but you do it in your own way, there is no right or wrong way. It is your way and it is the way that is right for you...I want you to totally relax, and when I begin to take you on your journey I will place my hands about an inch above you and I will hold them above you at various points on your body. You may feel warmth coming from my hands, but that's okay, don't be worried by this, as I will never actually physically touch you. You might feel some odd sensations, or you might get tingles or numbness, but don't be worried by this as I will be working with your aura and your energies to heal you, and heal your spirit." I listened intently to my instructions and I felt suddenly very calm.

" You are walking along a path in the woods," she whispered.

And suddenly I was there, standing in the cool, dark woods. The trees were all shapes and colours but very tall, reaching up into the sunny blue sky, and they were intertwined with tangling ivy and some wore velvety jackets of moss. I could tell that the sky was sunny and blue as the woodland floor was dappled with patterns of dancing, lacy sunlight, which tiptoed over the leaves and the twigs and the little flowers of white and blue. There was a rich, earthy, peaty smell which was mixed with the heady smell of beautiful delicate bluebells and the thick rich smell of wild garlic, which spread out in merging marbling lakes of colour about my feet and all around as far as I could see. And silently they disappeared deep, deep into the depths of the forest, where the light dimmed and the old gnarled trees hugged each other for warmth. I began to follow the barky path through the woods, and as I brushed through the colourful carpet of garlic and bluebells they whispered out more of their beautiful strong smells as they bowed down politely and greeted me. And as I carried on walking along the path, I realised I could feel the soft bark and moss and leaves beneath my feet, and I realised that my feet were bare. And as I glanced down at myself I saw that I was wearing a flowing white cotton dress, all loose and billowing as I walked, and behind me my hair was loose and flowing and I could feel and smell beautiful wild flowers tucked behind each ear. The air was cool, yet I was warm, and a silence draped around the trees like a comfortable overcoat.

And as I continued to walk I was vaguely aware of a voice in the distance instructing me and guiding me on my journey, and as I went on my way the voice became a gentle hum and I could no longer hear the directions, I seemed to just somehow be aware of what I was doing and where I had to go.

At last the path broke through the edge of the protective woods and I was at the edge of a babbling, gently-flowing stream that twinkled and glittered as the sunshine danced on the top of the ripples. And across the stream was a little white wooden bridge, and my path led across it. I crossed over the arched bridge, and as I did I looked down and could clearly see the gentle stream flowing beneath my feet through the thick wooden slats. When I reached the other side I walked alongside the stream, following the path, as the sunlight shone brightly and the trees began to whisper and ruffle their leaves as the breeze skipped over and through them. And as I walked I became aware that I could hear something crunching underneath my feet, and I realised that my path had changed to smooth, creamy gravel along the bank of the stream. The grasses and reeds along the side of the bank were long and thickly pointing, and some were bent and bowed under their own weight, dabbling their fingertips in the stream as it softly swished by. My path then stopped at the edge of a long ranch fence, and where the path had stopped was a wooden stile, which I carefully climbed over into a lush green meadow. I could feel the cool grass under my feet and tickling between my toes as I walked through the field and up the grassy hill in front of me. There were wild flowers sprinkled all over the meadow that swept up the sides of the gentle hill in a kaleidoscope of colour. The sun was shining brightly, and I could feel its warmth caressing my skin as the gentle breeze rippled the hem of my skirt and gently brushed and teased my hair. All was completely peaceful except for the chirpy twitters of the birds announcing to all that the day was beautiful and all was well with the world. As I reached the top of the flowery hill I stopped and gasped open-mouthed at the amazingly wondrous and breathtaking views that stretched out into the distance and all around me. The hills and woods and streams seemed to roll on forever, there were no houses, no roads, no telegraph poles; just me, on a hill in the middle of God's most beautiful and wondrous creation. Once I had finished drinking-in the mesmerising beauty, I laid down in the cool fresh grass and shut my eyes. I could smell the freshness, hear the sweet-sounding birds, feel the warm sunshine on my face, and sense the gentle breeze lapping at my shores. When I opened my eyes again I saw above me a swarm of angry black balloons bobbing and straining to break free from the long black ribbons that held on to their tails and attached them securely to my left wrist. I stared up at them suddenly feeling sad, overwhelmed and slightly distressed, but by my right hand, lying in the cool grass was a large pair of glisteningly sharp scissors. I picked them up and held them tightly as I followed the first ribbon to the first balloon. And inside the first large, black, foul balloon I saw Dean, and all of the pain and hurt and anger and tears and fears that went with him. I concentrated on these thoughts and foul-stenched feelings until all of the thoughts and feelings that I had for him were captured, swirling in the murky mass underneath the taut skin of the black balloon. And once I was sure that all that was Dean was crushed into a ball and rolled up tightly inside it, I got my shining scissors and cut sharply through the black ribbon that bound all that was him to me. And as I lay on that beautiful, warm, sunny day, looking up at the sky and the balloons that blackly bobbed, I watched the first dirty, black, sinister balloon, bob and float and drift away, up and up and up and up until it had disappeared from sight and vanished. It was gone. Gone at last, gone for good, gone forever. And I lay there, still and calm, feeling a little bit lighter, and a little bit cleaner, as I eyed the remaining black, macabre balloons bobbing in the breeze. And I realised that each balloon that I saw bobbing menacingly above me contained one aspect or event or feeling which had driven me into the darkness. So slowly I checked each balloon over, one by one, making sure that every hurt and evil and pain and sadness was packed tightly into each and every one of them. Once I was really sure that the balloon was full with all that I wanted to be rid of, I would cut the cord and let it go, let it free, let it disappear for ever. And as I cut the ribbon on the last ball of blackness, and watched it disappear away, away, away, I felt light and clean and fresh and free. Totally free. I lay in the sunshine breathing in the fresh clean air, and soaking up the sun's rejuvenating energy, as the birds sang and my heart soared up and up into the bright blue sky. And when I was finally refreshed and totally ready, I got up slowly, and smilingly made my way back down the hill amongst the colourful sweet flowers. And as I went I picked an armful of the dazzlingly beautiful, radiant, rainbow flowers and filled my soul with their intoxicating perfumes. I climbed back over the stile, and meandered back along the path, over the arched white bridge and back into the protection of the old wise woods. And as I stood there amongst the trees, feeling warm, soothed, fresh and free, I smiled and smiled as I had not felt as happy as this for ages and ages and ages, for as long as I could remember. Then slowly I became aware of a gentle voice whispering through the trees.

"When you are ready open your eyes," it whispered. "Open your eyes."

I looked all around for the owner of the soft, soft voice, as I placed the bouquet of beauty at my feet and watched it softly splay and scatter its colours all around me, then I scrunched my eyes tightly shut. And as I opened them again I found myself laying flat on the table, back in the small plain room with Rosa, clutching a handful of bright shiny pebbles.

"Okay?" she asked, smiling. I nodded as I blinked and blinked and reacquainted myself with this new reality.

"You were very good at that. You are very open and very, very receptive. I could see your eyelids flickering and your eyes moving madly behind your lids as soon as you began your journey. Well done! Now sit yourself up very slowly as you might feel a little light headed." I concentrated hard on her face and what she was saying as I felt a little disorientated and then I felt an unexplainably odd sensation in my body. As I lay there I felt as though all of my aura and energy had sunk into the bottom half of my body, and all across the top of my body, my tummy and top halves of my arms and legs was a light and empty feeling, and everything was prickling with pins and needles. I sat up slowly and felt my energy rush around and back in to fill the spaces and gaps as it tried to get everything working properly again. It took a few minutes for my tingling body to shake itself back to normal, and as I waited I checked the time on my watch and to my amazement realised that I had been on my magical journey for nearly an hour. I couldn't believe that it had passed so quickly.

"I've done a lot of work on healing your energies so everything should feel much better now and your energy will be flowing freely as it should. You were right, though; you had a huge grey shadowy energy on and all around your right shoulder. It was hard to shift, but it has gone now. I think it had been there for quite a long time." For as long as I could remember, I thought.

"You may feel your energy return strongly to you tomorrow, or it may take a couple of weeks to adjust itself, but you will definitely feel it, and you will recognise it and know when it has happened, and it will make you feel much, much better," she explained.

"Thank you, that was wonderfully relaxing, I really enjoyed it, thanks so much," I said as I collected my things and made my way to the door.

"I really hope it works," I smiled as I said my goodbyes.

"I'm sure it will," Rosa smiled knowingly. Her eyes twinkling as I walked out of the door and into the real sunlight outside; and as I felt its real warmth caress my face, I smiled.

CHAPTER NINETEEN

The late Summer sun shone brightly through the streaky window and danced across the dust which gently and lazily rested on the windowsill. It seemed to me that it had quietly gathered there as time had slowly slipped by without me even realising, and that each fine layer showed me one month that had passed since I first came here to the unit, and there seemed to me to be at least five layers sitting there waiting. Waiting for me to get better. A dusty calendar marking the passing of time, and quietly waiting for the moment for me to wipe it away, and for someone else to take my place, and watch their own dust settle. I felt deep down that it would soon be time to bring my duster and polish with me, and for me to finally wipe my slate clean.

I sat in the so familiar chair clutching my letter to Guy, and the one and only small photo that I had of him. Sylvia took the photo gently from my hand.

"So this is Guy then," she smiled, finally being able to place a face to the name she had heard so often. "It doesn't help does it, him being quite this handsome."

"No," I whispered trying to return her smile, but finding it hard. Writing the letter and digging out the photo left me feeling as if I had poured a cellar full of salt into a very open and very raw wound. The pain was searing and very, very real. She put the photograph onto the table, sat back in her chair and her eyes returned to me.

" Would you like to read the letter to me or would you like me to read it myself?" she asked. I sat up tall and strong in my chair and told her that I wanted to read the letter to her, it was my thoughts and feelings and recollections and I wanted to express them fully. I unfolded the thick wad of paper in my hand, took a deep, deep breath and began to read.

Dear Guy,

Well here I am, sitting here thinking about you and the wonderful relationship that we had, or at least I thought we had until I saw the reality of what was really there. The trouble was I saw it too late didn't I? Too late to be able to stop the damage. Anyway, let me begin at the beginning. I was sitting in the bar with my friend Anna, and we saw you and we both commented on how you were good looking for an older bloke. She couldn't believe it when I rang her two days later and told her we were going out on a date. I couldn't believe it myself to be honest, but we went out and we had a fantastic time. We couldn't stop laughing, and it seemed like we had known each other for years and years we got on so well. I remember ringing my mother up after that first date and telling her that I knew that you were the man I was going to marry. I was so, so sure. I wish I hadn't felt like that though. I wish I had seen through your bubbly effervescent exterior to the complete bastard that you were, but I couldn't. Or maybe I just didn't want to. Underneath that muscular frame, thick grey hair and charming smile you were a complete shit, and I was blind. Totally blind. After only six weeks you asked me to marry you, we chose a ring and you said that you were going to take me out, make me feel special, treat me like a queen, and ask me properly. So on the night when it was all to happen I got myself ready and I was really, really excited. You came and picked me up, but instead of a romantic restaurant you took me to some grotty, shabby place. I was so disappointed. You were always boasting about how much money you had and how much money you earned from your 'really important' television cameraman's job. So I expected romance and flowers and champagne, but I got a grotty cafe and a hurried unromantic proposal, and that was that, like it or lump it. I couldn't believe my eyes; after I had said yes, stupidly, you got up and left me on my own to go and talk to some woman that you hadn't seen for years at the bar. You left me sitting there like a complete fool on what was supposed to be the most romantic night of my life, and the waitresses clucked around me and tutted at your thoughtlessness. I was so, so embarrassed. And as I sat and looked at the ring sparkling on my finger a cold, scared feeling tugged at my stomach, somewhere deep inside, but I ignored it. This was wonderful, this was exciting, this was romance! But actually this was shit. You worked away during the week, and at weekends I would go and stay with you. Things seemed wonderful. You said you liked the thought of me being in your house and waiting for you while you were away, and I wanted to be closer to you, so I moved in, even though it meant leaving my cat behind. Sophie was looked after by my lodger, and I went back nearly every day to check on her and everything seemed fine. So there I was, in your house, doing what you wanted. It had begun hadn't it? The takeover. Then your son began to visit every other weekend. This was the first time I had met him as you hadn't been allowed to see him for six months. Something to do with your ex-wife's crazy accusations, and you told me it was because you were refusing to pay her money, and that was why she was saying the things that she did. I asked you why you had got divorced. You said she divorced you on the grounds of 'unreasonable behaviour'. I can understand it now, it's all so clear. Anyway Steven came down to stay, and he was a completely spoilt brat. I had worked with hundreds of different children through a range of ages, but I can honestly say I had never come across such a weird and spoilt relationship. I tried to talk to you about it so many times, but we always ended up rowing. "How the hell do you know anything about children, you'll never know about children until you have one of your own!" you'd say, knowing all the time that I might not be able to have any of my own. You loved to twist the knife didn't you. Of course you having him for two days out of fourteen meant you knew more about children than me having a class full of them for ten days out of fourteen. You knew everything, and I knew nothing, as always. As always you were right and I was always wrong. I wasn't allowed to ask him to do a single thing, I wasn't allowed to tell him off, I wasn't allowed to say or do anything without your permission, not even when we were living together and he was in 'our' home. It tore me to bits, but you just didn't care did you? Anything to keep 'Stevie-poo' happy wasn't it? You wanted to make him like you more than he liked his mother didn't you, and you did whatever it took, at the expense of everything and everyone around you. You were completely obsessed weren't you? I counted thirty-six photos of him around the house when I first met you. I thought it was odd but I never said anything. Just like I gave up trying to point out to you that it was unnatural for you to still share a bath with him when he was eleven years of age, and just like it was unnatural for you to share the bed with him and not me when he came to stay. I know you wanted to be close to him but this was ridiculous. You just didn't want to know; you just would not listen. Your way was right. It would eat me up inside every time he came down, as long as you had him you didn't want to know me. I tried so hard to join in, so hard to be part of our part-time family, but you hated it didn't you? You hated me because I was trying, so every time I tried you would find fault and criticise. If I tried I was wrong, and if I didn't try I was wrong. I played football with you, went boating with you, went to the cinema with you, tried so hard to make it work, but you didn't want it to did you? Not really. You wanted to completely dominate him, and you wanted to completely dominate me. I used to hate it when you would take him to your mother's house, just across town, so she could see her grandson. You never took me though, did you? I didn't exist as far as she was concerned. You told me that she still thought you were married to Karen. You had been divorced for six years; didn't you think that it was a bit odd and that you were a bit weird? I thought you were. What was wrong with me, was I not good enough, not pretty enough, or were you just ashamed of me? Or was there some other reason, some other dark secret that you were keeping from me? For the whole of the time that I was with you I never met or never spoke to anyone in your family, not your mother, two sisters or two brothers. Why not? You never even got a birthday card or Christmas card from any of them, what the hell had you done? What had gone on? It just didn't seem right to me. Alarm bells began to quietly ring, but I muffled them with my stupidity.

You hated the relationship I had with my family too didn't you? You did everything to try and slyly cause upset and arguments. You hated it when my parents rang me and you would stand there right next to the phone and listen and glower over me until I put the phone down, which I always did quickly because I couldn't cope with the pressure of it. I couldn't ring them that often, because I knew you checked the phone bill that you had had itemised specially, and you got angry if I did. In fact you would quiz me about all of the numbers on there that you didn't recognise wouldn't you. Just to check I wasn't having that imaginary affair that you thought I was having. You hated me visiting my family too. I was wrong if I joined in with you and Steven, I was wrong if I didn't join in with you and Steven, and I was wrong if I suggested I went to see my family as an alternative. It was really difficult knowing that everything I ever said or did would always be wrong. You were determined to destroy the relationship I had with them though weren't you? You would always pull me in the opposite direction to them, and you had a wonderful way of making me feel like I had done something bad and made me feel incredibly guilty every time I had any contact with them. I felt like my heart was being torn in two, and that made you really happy didn't it?

I remember when we went to visit the vicar to arrange our wedding. I remember sitting there getting more and more embarrassed as the whole of the time you were there you talked about you and Karen and the divorce and Steven. Never once did you mention me, never once did you mention why it was that we were getting married or what you felt for me. The final straw came when the vicar asked you if we wanted any children. And you replied, 'Oh yes, Stevie has always wanted a little brother or sister.' What about me, what about what I wanted, what about us? No, all you cared about was getting one over on Karen, she hadn't given 'Stevie-poo' what he wanted so you wanted to make sure that you did first. What were you going to do if I couldn't have children? Divorce me and find someone who could? Who knows. Anything was possible in your sick and twisted world. You could never fathom out why I was upset that day could you? You never could.

We spoke about selling both of our houses and moving into a cottage in the countryside, a dream come true for me. So we put our houses on the market, strangely enough you made me sell mine, but then decided not to sell yours. 'We'll wait for a while,' you said. And as for all of my furniture and everything that I owned? Well I had to get rid of it all didn't I! None of it was any good was it, according to you, none of it was better than anything that you had so it all had to go. All I had in 'our' house were my clothes, books, some bits and bobs in the kitchen, cassettes and the cat – which you despised. I had a washing machine that was banished to the garage as it wasn't as good as yours despite it being five years younger, so mine was 'oops, sorry, dropped it,' on the way to the garage to ensure it wasn't used, and my bed which was also banished to the garage as it was 'much too uncomfortable.' Funny how they were both good enough for you to try and sell behind my back once I had moved out.

So there I was, trapped in the house with you, your things, your part-time son, and your vile temper and childish ways. From then on everything I did, or didn't do was wrong. I had to grow my hair longer, had to grow my fringe out, had to go blonde. So I did what I thought would make you happy, I couldn't cope with the ridicule. My clothes were always wrong, totally wrong. So I wore what you told me I could, it saved a lot of fuss and upset didn't it? I was kind of spooked when I found your secret stash of Karen photos, 'they're for Stevie-poo,' you said. I wasn't convinced, I was just scared. As I stared at the photos the woman that stared back looked a lot like me, just her hair was longer and blonder; I was getting there though wasn't I? But in your eyes I would never get anything right. You taught me my morning routine didn't you, I was very grateful. I had to get up and pull the curtains first, then I had to make the bed before I left the bedroom. None of this 'have a shower first', I had to open the curtains and make the bed in that order; it wasn't worth my while to do anything different was it? Once I had finished getting dressed I had to make sure that the toilet seat was down, the shower curtain was drawn correctly and that all of the upstairs doors were shut before I could come downstairs. Had to get it right, had to get it right. Then I had my clothes washing rules, obviously my washing machine and the powder that I bought were no good at all, so that all had to go. The clothes had to be washed in a certain way and I never managed to hang them on the line correctly did I? I never fathomed what it was that I did so terribly wrong, but I must have always been doing something wrong as I always got shouted at didn't I. When it was raining I would put the clothes on the radiators to dry, but I managed to get that wrong too and I used to make the house damp, apparently. Sorry, I forgot that I had to magically dry clothes with the power of my mind! My car was wrong too wasn't it? You hated the fact that I had bought it myself and that it was exciting and different to most of the cars around, so you kept on at me until I changed it to something conventional. The deciding factor came on the night it broke down, do you remember? It was a freezing cold, dark night and I broke down on the side of the motorway, and I was absolutely terrified. I had no phone so I got out in the cold and dark, and fought my way along the hard shoulder through the rain. Luckily someone I knew recognised the car and stopped, rang the AA then went on his way. When I got back to my car the police were there, so I sat in the car with them until the AA arrived. I had to go in the tow truck and take the car to my mechanic, and the kind AA man let me ring you on his phone to tell you what had happened as you had been expecting me to pick you up from the pub. When I called you, you were really cross with me and said it was my fault for having such a stupid car. Five minutes after I had put down the tow truck phone it started ringing. The man picked it up and it was you, wasn't it? I was so embarrassed because you began to scream and scream at me down the phone, "Why the hell were you with that friend who rung the AA? Are you having an affair with him?" you screamed. I couldn't believe my ears, I was scared, I was cold, and I was lucky enough to be spotted by my friend on the hard shoulder and all you could do was accuse me of having an affair with him, and you said I had spent the evening with him and that I had been lying to you. I couldn't believe it; I was so upset. You really didn't give a shit about me and how I was, you just wanted to scream and scream about me having this imaginary affair. You even accused me of planning to run away with him and said I had been planning this all along. I couldn't believe my ears. I was stunned, upset, and completely humiliated. When I eventually got home, four hours late, way after midnight, I was really chuffed to think that you had waited up for me, waited to see if I was okay after my really upsetting ordeal, but you hadn't had you. You screamed at me for having an affair, screamed at me for planning to run away from you, and once I had convinced you that you were talking rubbish you screamed at me for not picking you up from the pub on time. I had broken down, been in a police car, been in a tow truck for hours, been miles away to my mechanic to drop the car off, been scared, and cold and worried and upset and all you could do was scream about me not picking you up from the pub on time! What the bloody hell was I supposed to do?! I was stunned by your reaction, and your twisted mind certainly showed its true colours that night. You harassed me about my car so much after that, I actually changed that too. But when my new one arrived at the garage, and I got really excited about it, do you remember, you refused to take me to pick it up. It sat there for a week before you would take me down to collect it. You were such a shit. If I had a smile on my face you would do your best to scrape it off wouldn't you. You were sickly perverse and a total bully. You took all of your own inadequacies out on me and it just wasn't fair. You were so, so cruel. So cruel; I couldn't really believe the things that you did and said, and all that was going on around me. I just couldn't understand it at all.

You didn't like me having friends either, did you? You didn't like them ringing the house, or coming to visit, in fact you were so rude to them when they did ring up that they all eventually stopped ringing. I was quite relieved in a way as I couldn't cope with you standing there and listening to my every word, and I couldn't cope with the rows afterwards. You were happy then, weren't you, you shit? You didn't have any real friends, so you didn't want me to have any either. But still I refused to see the truth. Actually I think deep down I did see the truth but I refused to acknowledge it. I didn't want to admit I had cocked it up yet again, and I couldn't face the reality that I had nowhere to go, had nothing left, had no-one to turn to, you had made sure of that hadn't you? Destroying everything that I had, and then beginning to destroy me bit-by-bit, drop-by-drop. My self-esteem had always been low, but you managed to smash it completely to bits. I hate you, you complete and utter bastard. What a clever game you played.

We began to make wedding plans didn't we? Well I began to make wedding plans didn't I? You really weren't interested, were you? And you'd shout at me every time I tried to get you to come with me to choose something. You even caused a big row about going to book the venue; you just wanted to spoil every thing I tried to do. I kept asking you if you were sure that you still wanted to get married, I didn't mind if you didn't want to, I just didn't want to book all of these things and spend all of this money if you were unsure. I didn't want to marry anyone who was unsure. But you kept telling me you loved me and it was what you wanted, despite your actions that said otherwise. Two months before it was due to happen we, (well you, actually) decided that we should postpone the wedding indefinitely as we were having problems. I had to agree as things were getting worse and worse between us, and you were messing more and more up inside my head. It was funny really, you, sorry 'we', called the wedding off but you made me face the humiliation and the upset of cancelling everything alone. And I was the one who had to pay all of the lost deposits back to my father. I lied and told him you had paid, but I think deep down he knew it was me. You thought it was all pretty amusing didn't you, seeing me upset, humiliated and lying. I had to cancel the church, the vicar, the cars, the reception, the band, the catering, the cake, the photographer, the flowers, sort the dress out, and I had to pay for and collect the box of invitations, pretending everything was fine and rosy to the excited shop assistants when they asked me all about the 'big day'. Inside my heart was breaking, and you thought it was all good sport, you were such a bastard, sitting there all the time, grinning and grinning and grinning in your smug controlling way. I don't think you were ever going to go through with it; it was just a big funny game to you. By the time all of this happened you had destroyed all of the confidence that I had, all of the things that I had and everything that made me happy, you had poisoned. I couldn't say the right thing, I couldn't do the right thing, and inside I was in perpetual confusion and turmoil. I used to make sure that I cleaned the house every Thursday before you came home on the Friday, and I would always make sure that the fridge was full of things you liked, I had cooked a nice meal and that I had made myself look nice for when you got home on the Friday. I was so pleased to see you. How fucking stupid was I? You would come through the door, and you would criticise my cleaning, then you would criticise the food that I had bought, then you would criticise my cooking. Everything I did, and every time I tried to make you feel special you threw it back in my face. It got so bad that you told me when you came back on a Friday you wanted time to unwind on your own and you didn't want to see me until you were ready. So I would sit in the bedroom with my best clothes on and wait and wait and wait until you were ready to see me. I would sit there for hours sometimes, looking back I can see what a sick bastard you were, but at the time you had screwed my head up so much that I thought this was normal, I thought that that was all that I was worth. I could never argue with you about any of this as you would get so angry and explode so badly that I would be terrified, so in the end I couldn't fight back, I would just take it and take it and take it. I even remember on the Fridays that you went to collect Steven that I would stay on late at school so that I didn't get home before you and Steven did. I would stay so late that I would be thrown out by the caretaker, because I knew that if I got home before you both and made dinner, I would get it wrong, and if I got home before you both and didn't make dinner, it would also be wrong, so I decided hiding at school was easier. Even then I pretended to myself and all around that everything was okay. But it was not okay, something was seriously wrong and I was terrified.

I will never forgive you for the way that you treated me when Aaron and Nanny Joan died. You were heartless and selfish and downright cruel. And I hated you for it, hated you more than you will ever know.

It seemed that the more I crumbled, and the more ill that I got, the happier you were. It was easier for you to control me then wasn't it? And I was too stupid, confused, worn down and ill to realise it. It was terrible to watch, it seemed that you had a nuclear self-destruct button, which your finger was always caressing and hovering over. You couldn't believe that someone actually loved you as much as I did, and you were going to test and test and destroy and mangle it until you could say 'I told you so, you didn't really love me.' So you carried on sending me over and over, harder and harder emotional assault courses.

I remember so many times sitting at the railway station not far from our house, crying and crying with my bags packed and wondering where the hell to go and what the hell to do, I just needed a break, just needed some time to think and to get away from you. But you never let me stay away for long did you, and I would always stupidly go back. My friends and family had all at some point had to pick me up from the station in a terrible state because of the things that you said and because of the things that you did. I remember the time that you screamed and screamed at me, I can't even remember what for now, but you screamed until I cried so much I thought my head would explode. Then you took Steven by the hand and went off, smiling and smiling, so smug that you had upset me, and you had blocked my car in the garage with your car and had taken the keys with you. Taken the keys so that I had to stay there, had to wait for you to come back and give me round two of the abuse. But I wasn't there when you got back was I? You thought I was trapped, but I wasn't. I had gone to my favourite place, the station, and been picked up by my grandmother, so that I could at least have a bit of a break from the torrent of abuse. And sometimes I would just get onto a train, any train, and go away, away, away to think, away from you so that I could even breathe.

By the time we reached Christmas I didn't know what I was doing, where I was going, what I wanted or even who I was at all. I couldn't think anymore, I couldn't feel anymore and my life was falling apart in lumps, and all the time you smiled. I remember Christmas Day, even though I was malfunctioning. You bought me a bike, the one you wanted so that you could use it, and a dress. I had to wear the dress, I had no choice, I was a dolly for you to dress up. So I painted on my smile and you took me to your friend's house and dangled me in front of them like the puppet that I was, and I performed on command, as I had learnt to do so well. Once I had received a round of applause you took me home, and then ignored me. So I slumped in the corner, as you were bored with your Christmas toy, and waited for my next instruction. I don't remember you speaking to me again that day as I had fulfilled my role, and like a good little girl was seen and not heard, and did everything that I was told. And you had been your usual glorious bastard self."

I stopped.

"I didn't write any more," I said red faced and so, so angry. "I stopped because I realised as I was writing and writing that I had had so much of my life and so much of my time destroyed and infected by him that I didn't want to waste one more second thinking about him. It's over. It _is_ all over."

I had felt such a great sense of triumph and such a great sense of control when I had stopped writing. I realised that I was angry with myself – angry with myself at letting him dominate yet more of my time, and it was time to stop. Now I was the one in control.

I carried on telling Sylvia about what then happened, so that I could finally tie up the loose ends of the tale, and finally gain the closure that my heart and mind demanded.

My life had turned into a living nightmare and I was a prisoner inside its poisonous bars. I had lost my home, I had lost my belongings, I had lost my friends and I was not allowed to see my family without permission. I was completely controlled, and I could see no way out of the mess that I found myself in. Everything I said was wrong, everything that I did was wrong, everything that I didn't say was wrong and everything that I didn't do was wrong. I was continually wrong, and continually bombarded with the abuse that comes with being permanently wrong. I doubted everything that I said, and I doubted everything that I did, until I didn't know what I was doing and I didn't know who I was anymore. It was as if I had to ask permission to even be able to think. I spent the whole time in terrified inaction like a rabbit staring into the headlights of a car, never knowing which way to turn, never knowing just what to do. The continual undermining, ridicule and mental abuse ate away everything that made me me. And why did I stay with him? Well it was that strangely stupid thing that masqueraded as love. I sometimes wished that he had hit me. It would have been easier if he had hit me. "If anyone ever hit me that would be it," I would say, it would have been the excuse, the trigger that would have made me get up, hold my head high and leave him. But mental abuse was different. How can you define what it is, how it works, and how it slowly but surely completely destroys you? It starts quite small to begin with, and you pass it off as just one of those things, and then it gets worse and worse and worse until you don't know which way is up and which way is down and your head turns inside out in your unrecognisable world of pain. I wanted a sign, I wanted someone to tell me when enough was enough and at what point I should walk away in order for me to save my sanity. But that point never came. I never knew when it was time to go, as by the time I realised that that point had come it was too late, far too late. I had been destroyed and I was too helpless to help myself.

He had destroyed everything in my life and he had been destroying everything inside my head. And the more he destroyed inside my head the less able I was to see a way out, less able to think about what I could do. My head swam permanently with fog, my heels dragged as I walked, and even breathing became an effort. My mind spun in pointless never-ending circles and the darkness swooped in with its big black cloak and smothered me until it was so densely black in the darkness that I could no longer see. I would walk the streets in the rain with my head spinning, and think to myself that I couldn't live with him anymore as he was smashing me to pieces, but I couldn't live without him as I had nothing left, no-one to turn to, and in my distraught state I still believed that I loved the monster that was him. I couldn't live with him, and I couldn't live without him. The only way out that I could see was the dark way out, the sad way out, the coward's way out. I toyed with the idea of plunging into death and the hows and the wheres and the consequences it would have on those around me.

I was so drained of every drop of energy that I had, as I had used it all up in the endless struggling fight, that dying was the only welcoming, calm, sweet option that I could see. And each day I battled with the gentle blackness that beckoned me with her delicate bony finger, as she whispered promises of warmth and love, stillness and peace. She looked so beautiful as she stood in the shelter and smiled, and I stood outside as the tempestuous hurricane swirled and smashed, and the vicious rain pelted like splintering sheets of glass, which sliced and shredded my skin until my heart and soul bled, my life drained away, and I stood there, the ghost that once upon a time had been me.

On the last night, after he had shouted and screamed and swore and ranted so much that I lay in bed alone with my migraine, alone with my sadness, alone with my tears and my fears, I heard a voice. A voice from somewhere deep, deep inside me, and it whispered to me through the thick tarry blackness and the swirling storm, and it told me it was now time to go. I lifted the receiver of the phone that sat on my bedside table and rang my mother.

"I'm coming home." I whispered, as the tears gently rolled down each side of my face and dampened the pillow under my head. She understood. She always did. The next day, when I had gathered the little strength that I had and found myself alone in the house,

I got my suitcase and packed as much as I could carry, and walked away. I told him I just needed a break, but in my heart I knew I could never go back. If I did, it would kill me. Literally. We kept in contact for as long as it took me to get my cat, and eventually, when he had realised that he had lost the fight, my things. He begged and begged and begged, but I knew if I went back I would never be able to leave him again. The pain I felt inside was crucifying, but through the tangled spinning mess inside my head I knew it was the only way. It hurt like hell but if something is gangrenous and about to kill you, you have to cut it off and not mourn its loss.

He had carried on calling me, even after I had collapsed at school and been signed off from work. And as I was so ill I found I could not muster the strength to finally say no to him, and let it all go. On the day that I finally actually admitted to myself that I was very seriously ill, I knew I could never speak to him or see him again, and I used all of the strength that I had to make sure that I never did see him or speak to him again. And when we moved house, I made sure he never knew where I went. And I made sure that in moments of weakness that I didn't ring him up and open the slowly healing wound once more. It was not easy, but I would never give in.

I looked up at Sylvia. It was all finally over. And I began to realise that I would never understand why he was the way that he was, or why he did the things that he did, and I was determined I was not going to waste one more second of my precious life trying to fathom the unfathomable. I was finally ready to let go. We went into the office and Sylvia enlarged the photograph onto ten sheets of paper with the photocopier and led me to the shredding machine, then smiling at me she turned it on.

"Go on," she said gently. "Let it go."

I stood trembling at the whirring, grinding, grinning teeth, with my letter and the photographs in my hand, and began to let it all go.

"Good-bye..." I whispered, as I watched his face disappear time and time again, and watched it tumble out of the machine like cleansed confetti. And finally, as my last tears traced my cheeks, I pushed my angry words and angry feelings and pain and hurt and all consuming raging anger into the mouth of the cleansing machine, and finally I felt complete. Resolved, cleansed, complete. I was finally free, I was finally me, and I was finally ready to begin facing the world. It was over. It was all over. I was free. Free in every way imaginable.

It seemed funny as I blinkingly walked out into the warm sunshine with my bucket of pebbles. Everything suddenly seemed much brighter.

CHAPTER TWENTY

I sat and eyed the all-important stories in the local weekly newspaper (the all-important stories to the locals, and the completely unimportant stories to the rest of the world). I suppose it's human nature, the things that are important, that affect us and that influence the way that we think, the way that we react and the way that we live our lives, are things that are completely meaningless and unimportant to other people. Sometimes I found it mind-boggling to think of how many people there were living in a street, and how many people there were living in that town, and how many people there were living in that country, and how many people there were living in the whole of the world, and how each individual person was living their own life in their own way with their own ideas, lifestyle, experiences and problems. Millions of people, and yet each and every one of them was unique, and each and every one of them was alone. And all of these people were living in a world where even their next-door neighbour didn't know what they were thinking or doing or feeling. And I thought if even their neighbour didn't know these things, then how could we ever understand the thoughts and the lives and the feelings of someone living in the next street, the next town, the next country? I always wondered about people, and the lives they might be living, the things they might be doing, and the relationships they might have as I watched them shuffling along the street with their grey faces and their grey clothes living their grey lives. I would wonder what went on behind the scenes, and behind their grey masks, and I would wonder what it was all about, each person side-by-side but unique and so very alone. Alone and not understanding, or indeed even knowing their neighbour, or knowing anything about anyone else's lives, or feelings or thoughts. Everybody was so, so alone. And once I had finished thinking about all of these millions and billions of people all living their own lives with their own thoughts and their own feelings in their own way I would think that all of these people were connected in some way and in fact everyone in the world had a connection with everyone else in the world. I had this idea that if you took one person and knocked on every door in a street eventually that person would meet someone he knew. Then if those two people carried on knocking on doors they would find someone else that one of them knew. Then if those three people carried on knocking they would find someone else that one of them knew. And if they carried on, and collected each person that one of them knew, eventually they would end up collecting everyone in the whole wide world. So everyone did indeed have a connection with everyone else in the whole world, and it would do them well to remember this when they were chopping down rainforests, or polluting the ocean, or mugging some old lady. They were hurting themselves as much as the people that they were affecting, as they were all joined together by some invisible force, some invisible thread. Sometimes my mind got carried away with itself. Sometimes I thought just too much. So I carried on reading the newspaper.

I read some of the stories in the paper that caught my eye, and looked with interest at the photos of some of the couples who had got married that week in the local churches and registry offices. I often chuckled at the various choices of dresses and headdresses and flowers and puffs and lace and fluff. Sometimes I couldn't believe that these people actually thought they looked okay in what they had chosen to wear. I also found that sometimes the couples looked extremely odd together, but they were always smiling, so they must be happy with each other, and indeed love each other in order for them to have got married in the first place. I often wondered what it was that people saw in each other, and what that magical thing was that made people fall in love. Or fall in what they thought was love.

My mind wandered again. I flicked through the 'What's on' guide, and the odd items for sale that the people no longer wanted or had room for in their lives. Then I turned to the jobs page. I always had a look at the jobs page to see what was about and what other people were doing with their lives. Not looking for a job for myself, just inquisitive. There were the usual care assistant jobs, cleaners, order pickers and factory workers, and then at the bottom of the page I spotted a tiny little advert.

'Part-time animal carer required at busy pet hotel. No experience necessary.'

That's interesting, I thought to myself. I had worked at a cattery for four years while I had been at school, at weekends and school holidays, and I had really enjoyed it. I turned the advert over in my mind. Over and over and over. 'Maybe I could do this,' I thought. It was only part-time, so I could still have time to sleep during the day and still have time to write, and it was a job working with animals, which I loved. You don't have to report to animals, you don't have to take orders from them, if they like you they lick you, wag their tail or purr, and if they don't like you they bite you – simple as that. You know exactly where you are with them. And I thought to myself, 'why don't you give it a try? It will give you something to focus on, you will enjoy working with the animals and if you can't cope you can walk out, it won't matter, it won't affect anyone and at least you will have tried.' And before I had time to think about what I was talking myself into and the prospect of getting the job and feeling the fear of what I may possibly be about to embark upon, I found that I had rung the telephone number on the advert and was talking directly to the boss. After a long chat he asked me to come in the next day and see how I got on.

I slumped in the chair. Shocked, stunned, flabbergasted. What had I done? I chuckled to myself, 'you are definitely bonkers!' I thought.

Mum came in through the front door with her hands full of bags of bulky groceries, looking tired and a little harassed after a day at work. I took some of the bags from her and began helping to unpack the fruit and the veg and the tins of this and that.

"Mum," I said, shaking a little and laughing at myself for doing something so daft, "I've got a job."

She dropped her bags of shopping on the floor; luckily I had already packed the eggs away.

I told her what had happened and that I thought the least I could do was try. It was no pressure, no hassle, no stress and I could walk away if things got too much. She was dumbfounded, but extremely happy. She said she thought it was a wonderful idea, as long as I thought I could really cope with it, and she said she was very proud of me for at least being brave enough to give it a go. I was really pleased she was proud of me, as I was going from being a teacher to a poo-shoveller, but she said if it made me smile then she didn't care what it was that I was doing. I could be a stuntwoman, a road sweeper, or a trapeze artist for all she cared, as long as I was smiling.

I got up nice and early the next day, and the sun streamed in through the crack in the curtains and danced across the ripples of the cream duvet. I put on my oldest faded blue jeans, an old black t-shirt saved especially for dirty jobs, and a pair of black wellies that I had managed to dig out from the depths at the back of the garage, and summoning up all of my strength, off I went in my little red car. Mum and Dad waved me off and wished me good luck as I drove away. I was sure they were more nervous and worried than I was. I could see it etched heavily across my mother's face, and upon my father's forehead hung a wrinkly frown. They were brilliant. They worried themselves to death about me but were so very supportive, through everything I was going through, and through everything that I had put them through.

My little car weaved its way along the hedge-lined lanes through the expanse of flat and even fields. The spiders webs glistened from the morning dew and were decked with decadent diamonds as they draped over each and every branch and hedge. I drove through the small creamy-stoned village, with its obligatory school, post office and pub, and saw the postman delivering his news that made you smile or made you cry or made you go reaching for your bank statement to check if what you're reading could possibly be true. As I came out of the little village the lane began to get narrower and wound its way up high into the tree-topped hills in front of me. The cottages became sprinkled further and further apart and were replaced by the occasional farmhouse dotted amongst the waving crops, the cows, the sheep, the trees and the empty fields ready and waiting for their next role. I carried on wiggling along the tiny lane and eventually came to a small tarmac parking area coming off the lane. Along the wall beside the parking area were garishly painted cartoon pictures of cats and dogs in silly poses doing silly things like hang gliding and skate boarding and were all grinning foolishly. 'Mmm,' I thought, 'how tasteful.'

I parked the car, opened the big green metal gates and walked into the grounds of the huge kennels and cattery. A large, red-faced man with a fuzz of blond hair greeted me, and he seemed to me to be in his early fifties. He looked rather jolly and was wearing an enormous pair of green wellies, brown trousers, and a bright yellow top, and he welcomed me heartily with a firm and sticky handshake. He began by showing me around the kennels. We walked past caged outdoor run after caged outdoor run of barking, sleeping, bouncing, eating, pooping, playing dogs, from the size of a small hairy rat to an enormously large and gangling, slobbering, donkey-sized creature. I was no good with breeds. Then I realised, oh my God! I had never even walked a dog before! But each different face greeted us with excited glee, and despite the ear-splintering barking commotion, they all made me smile. We walked along the inside rows of sleeping compartments, where their blankets and toys had been piled into their beds ready for them to throw around in excitement again. And each little face that had greeted us on the outside rampaged and bounced and staggered and wandered into each of their bedrooms, and barked and smiled at us on the inside. There was an overwhelming smell of all things dog and a hint of cleaning chemicals. We then went to the more civilised end of the market, the cattery. They too had their inside bedrooms where they lazed in their multicoloured fluffy beds, and their outside caged runs, where they sprawled on the sun decks or went cleanly and conveniently to the loo in their litter trays. Well most of the time anyway. Some of them were nervous and huddled underneath their upturned bed, confused, upset and waiting for some kind of reassurance from someone, anyone. Some of them sat outside and eyed the rabble of dogs in the distance, with a disdainful look of disgust upon their elegant and far superior faces. Some of the younger cats rolled on the floor in the sunshine, with a tufty toy mouse, a cotton reel or a ping pong ball, all practising their hunting skills for that time, one day in the future, when they might actually be able to capture something for themselves. But mostly the black and the white and the tabby and the tortoiseshell creatures lounged and laid and sprawled and snored curled up or stretched out in their own little beds. I knew they found it hard to survive with less than twenty-three hours sleep a day. And I knew how that felt. It was so much cleaner and brighter, less smelly and far more sophisticated than the dog accommodation. But I should have expected it, they were cats after all, and cats demand nothing but the best.

I didn't get to work with the cats on that first day, but I did receive my baptism of fire with the motley crew of dogs. First we had to walk them, so I was shown the ropes by Kate. She was a young twenty-something, also in a yellow top, and she had tied up her long dark hair behind her head, for two reasons, she told me. The first was to avoid dangling it into various unmentionables, and secondly to avoid someone deciding to play 'raggie' with it and dragging her playfully around the kennel by it. She was friendly and happy and we got on rather well. She showed me how to put a lead on a dog and how to work the safety doors. Then she explained how we walked the dogs around the paddock every morning. To let them stretch their legs and to let them go to the loo; less for us to clean up in the kennels I was told. How delightful. So there I was, full of fear and trepidation, standing outside the run of the first dog I was to walk. I looked suspiciously at him, and he sat dopily and wagged his old knobbly tail at me. I stood and I made my decision there and then that I was not going to be scared, I was going to be confident, I was going to be calm, and I was going to be in control. Dogs sense fear, and I was going to lose before I even went in with them if I was hesitant and unsure. So I opened the door and strode right on in, and with my best Oscar-winning performance of confidence, making out it was the most natural thing in the world, I pretended that I had done it thousands of times before. The little black boy looked up at me with his big soft dark eyes, and he wagged his tail happily from side to side. He was a little Labrador cross and he had a delightfully speckly, grey, old man's muzzle. I put on the lead and led him out onto the paddock. We wandered together, at his geriatric pace, and he sniffed the bushes and the flowers as we passed by, and occasionally he did some of his business. He was so, so cute as he shuffled along, and he seemed so pleased to be with me. Herbie melted my heart, and when I put him back we had a huge cuddle and he licked my face. I had made a friend. I made lots of friends that morning: bouncing, boisterous boxers that dragged me around the paddock, trampolining on me at every opportunity; burstingly happy, waggy and friendly golden retrievers, which loved you to bits and usually brought you one of their toys or their blanket in their mouth, to say thank you or to try and bribe you to stay; looney and boingingly clumsy chocolate Labradors who thought it was fun to bounce up to see you, nearly removing your front teeth with their thick heads as they did; little Yorkies that dangled on the end of the lead, making you almost forget that the little 'rats on a rope' were there. But they were excellent cuddling size; and West Highland Whites that marched you around the paddock, convincing you that they were at least eight foot tall and if they had their way would make a bid for world domination. There were big ones and small ones, bouncy and calm ones, old ones and young ones, scared and playful ones, and ones that were just not sure. And they dribbled and pooped and weed and bounced and licked and dragged and kicked mud and grass around, but they were all pleased to see me, even though the less confident ones needed gentle coaxing and TLC, and the psychotic springy ones needed firm but kind handling. And each moment I spent with them, and gave them love and attention, and got bounced on and licked and dribbled on, they gave me so much more back. I could feel a warm, happy, glow inside, and so, so much love. I felt like I was doing something worthwhile, I was making them feel safe and happy and loved and reassured, and they, in their hairy smelly way, were giving me all that they had back in return. I learnt about where things were, what to do, and how to feed them, and most importantly how to clean up the smelly messes that they left behind, or bounced delightfully in to, then on to you. But as I set to work armed with a bucket and a shovel, disinfectant and a brush, I smiled to myself. Luckily my stomach was strong and it didn't bother me at all. I was far happier shovelling it than having my life full of it, so that was fine by me.

At the end of the morning the jolly owner asked me how I felt about the job, how I got on, and whether I thought it was the right thing for me. And as I looked around at the rolling picturesque hills that spread out before me, and I looked at the row of waggy bottoms in the runs, and felt the sun blazing down on my face, I felt happy. Really, really happy. It was just the right job for me. Despite being dripping with sweat, stinking of dogs, feeling tired and mucky and having squelching soggy socks inside my wellies, I felt happy, like I had made a difference, like I had something to care for, and like something loved me back. And suddenly I felt like I was on top of the world. It might not be teaching, it might not be a career that I had aspired to, it might not be most people's idea of a sensible job, but I really didn't care. I had had the respected career, I had had the responsibility, I had used my skills and my intellect and did what I thought was supposed to be right, but I had been the most unhappy person in the world. And now I was smiling. And my heart was full of purpose and full of love. Many people turned their noses up when I told them that I had been a teacher, and now I was working in a kennels and cattery. What a let down, what a failure, what a disappointment. And then I would point out to them that the most important thing to me was that when I went to work I was smiling. And they would go away and think about the things that I had said, and then they began to realise that maybe I was not so crazy after all. And they all wished that they too carried a smile with them as they battled on the busses, with the people, in the traffic, in the fumes, with the drizzle. And the never-ending phone calls at the office and the backstabbing and the stress and the meetings and the rush, rush, rushing that they never seemed to escape from in the treadmill that was their lives. Yes, they too wished they carried a smile with them as they made their unhappy way to work. And I would ask them again, 'who was the mad one now?'

CHAPTER TWENTY-ONE

As I walked slowly up the crunchy gravel drive, with my package under my arm, I had a feeling deep inside that this might be the last time I would visit Sylvia at the mental health hospital. I don't know why, I just knew.

The sun shone brightly overhead, and the sky was the most brilliant blue shade that I could ever remember it being, and I wondered if anyone had ever found a sapphire as amazingly blue as that. I couldn't see a cloud anywhere, only the occasional white wisp of an angels breath, high, high up. The summer flowers were just hanging on to their last days of life, but were still radiantly beautiful and scattered in such a variety of colours they looked like a spilt bag of candy, and seemed just as sweet. And as I listened to the last twittery singing of the birds telling me of the exciting adventures they were about to embark upon, my eyes wandered up to the tall strong trees all around. I noticed that little tinges of yellow and orange and red were hiding amongst the greenery with their colourful little noses peeking out. Ready and waiting to rejuvenate themselves by sacrificing the old to make way for the fresh and the new. I was beginning to see so much more now, and I was beginning to feel alive.

The hospital had come to be a place of safety, a place of warmth and a place of cleansing, and it no longer filled me with the dread of knowing I was about to face my demons. It was a kind place, full of kind people, and it had come to be my safety blanket, my comforter. Here, everything would always end up being okay.

I sat in the little grey room, with my package placed under my chair. The windowsill had been cleaned, and the garden had replaced the dust and was hanging in the window like the most magnificent oil painting that I had ever seen. God was indeed the greatest artist of them all.

I found myself passionately telling Sylvia all about my new job, and how much I was enjoying it, and I told her all about the writing that I had done and how much I had enjoyed doing that too. Then I told her about how much more positive I had been feeling, and how I was even beginning to look forward to my unknown future. I wasn't sure if I was feeling good because of the counselling sessions, because of the medication, because of the spiritual healer, because of the love I had received from my family and friends or because of my own hard work. I think maybe it had been a little bit of all of them, and anyway it didn't matter which it was, it only mattered that I was feeling a whole lot better.

"Is there anything left that you would like to talk about?" she asked, smiling at the enthusiastic, shiny new person that sat before her. I frowned and thought, and thought, and thought, and deeply trawled inside my head, inside my heart and inside my soul, and after much searching I found that I had caught nothing. My nets were empty. And I too felt empty, confused, and a little bit lost, and then it began to dawn on me. I had nothing left to talk about. I had dredged and dredged, and sorted and washed and cleansed and thrown away all of the rubbish and debris and muck. And finally I realised that all I had left was myself, and an empty white new canvas that was ready for me to paint upon, ready for me to paint upon it pictures of my beautiful, new, happy life. And I would be the only person allowed to touch it and paint upon it, and nobody else would ever be allowed to touch it, not now, not later, not ever. No more blackness, no more dirt, no more putrid rotting. The black paint and the brushes of the demons had been thrown away, and they had been shattered for good.

And now I found myself sitting here feeling clean and light, but totally and utterly empty. I knew something was missing, but I couldn't quite put my finger on what it was. I suppose it was like someone who gives up a destructive habit like smoking, and they just don't know what to do with their hands anymore. Well it was a little bit like that. I had broken and got rid of all of the dirty black thought habits that had plagued me inside my head, and I now realised that I had to find new things to replace them. Nice thoughts, happy thoughts, creative thoughts. I had to start afresh, because there was no way I was going backwards. Sometimes people stick to the familiar, rather than face the unknown, no matter how bad or rotten the familiar may be for them, and no matter how much healthier it would be for them to stop and get rid of the bad things. They think that they just can't do it; that they're not strong enough or brave enough. They think it's far easier for them to bury their heads in the sand and carry on with the festering mess that is their life, rather than face an unknown and empty life without it. People just don't realise that they can fill that gap with whatever beauty and happiness they like, but to do this they have to do the difficult and painful thing, they have to make space for that happiness. And what they don't realise is that if they don't face their demons and devils, either in their heads or in their lives, they may one day not be able to face them at all, because they might just end up like I did. Only it might just be too late. No, I was not going to be like them, I would embrace the unknown and empty void left behind by the darkness that I had banished, and I would fill it with the life that deep down I had always truly wanted. I would fill the space with a life that was right for me. They may want to stay on the terrifying ride into the darkness on the worry-go-round, but I would never ride the bucking, kicking, black beasts again.

"I've got nothing left to talk about," I smiled brightly. "It's all finally gone. I don't need to talk about anything anymore as I think I've talked about just about everything."

I felt triumphant and exhilarated as we sat and chatted happily about the lovely things in life for a while, and then it was time for me to leave the session for the last time. We hugged as we said our goodbyes, and I felt a little pang of sadness as the door at the end of the corridor of now closed doors began to swing shut. It really was all finally over, and I felt bittersweet.

"Good luck with everything that you do," Sylvia spoke softly, "and remember that the door never closes for you here, it is always open."

I felt a little more reassured. She was the hand of my father on the back of my bike when my stabilisers were first taken off. Not really needed, but reassuring all the same.

"Thank you. Thank you for everything," I said, slightly choked and determined not to shed a tear.

"No, let me thank you," she said, to my surprise. "I have met many, many people in this job, but I can honestly say that I have never met anyone so doggedly determined to make themselves better. You did absolutely everything you could to beat this thing, and you surely and very successfully have." I was stunned, and inside I was swelling with pride. I knew she might well say this to everyone, but all the same I felt brilliant. I knew the fight was not over, and I knew that it may never be truly over but at least I had my own set of boxing gloves, just in case. But at that moment in time I didn't think about the possibility of relapses, or my impending battle to come off of the medication, because I knew in my heart I had already won the greatest battle of all. And as I held aloft my glittering trophy I drank in all of the happiness around me until I floated away in bubbly intoxication.

I wandered up to the florist and arranged for a beautiful lilac and mauve bouquet to be delivered to Sylvia. She had been wonderful and helped me struggle through the blackest and most frighteningly horrible experience of my life, and I wanted to thank her properly. It made me angry that people were often so quick to complain about things that were wrong, or when a service was inadequate, but it was very rare for people to ever show their appreciation and thanks for something that was good, or for someone who had worked incredibly hard on their behalf.

Before I had become ill I had always liked to make people smile, and the time had come to make people smile again. I wanted to make Sylvia smile, as she had spent so much time rekindling that long forgotten joy in me. And once I had chosen the flowers that I wanted to send to her, I wrote a little note to be sent with them,

'Dear Sylvia', it said, 'This is just a little way of showing you my thanks at you being there for me when I needed someone to talk to the most. I realise that it is your job to do this, but I am very grateful for everything that you have done. For listening, for supporting and for never ever judging the things that I told you, as so many people had done before. It takes a very, very special person to be able to do such a precious job as yours. And you are a very, very special person. I'll let you know how I get on in my brand new life, but for now I'll just send you all of my love and much, much thanks,

Rachael xx'.

I walked out of the shop and along the tree-lined road, where the sunshine still brightly shone and the birds still twittered sweetly, until I got to the small red post box. The post box that I had last used to post away my big black full stop. And here I stood again, fresh, clean, new, and so full of hopes and dreams my seams were now about to burst with happiness, and in my hand I held the thick heavy envelope. But this time it was a capital letter that I held so tightly, and I was ready to begin my new chapter. As I saw it disappear into the darkness with the same hollow plop, my dreams and memories went with it, and as I swam away I smiled. As pebble by hard-earned pebble I had rebuilt the dam of all things me, finally I was swimming in the beautiful warm waters of happiness, contentment and peace. And now I had learnt to swim I would never ever let myself drown again.